3-28-75

For Bob Michels

A reprint of one of the most popular books of the 19th century —

With best wishes,

Ted Carlson

The Constitution of Man Considered in Relation To External Objects

By George Combe

A Facsimile Reproduction
with an Introduction
By Eric T. Carlson, M.D.

Scholars' Facsimiles & Reprints   Delmar, New York, 1974

The Constitution of Man Considered in Relation To External Objects

By George Combe

A Facsimile Reproduction
with an Introduction
By Eric T. Carlson, M.D.

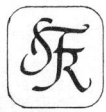

Scholars' Facsimiles & Reprints   Delmar, New York, 1974

Published by
Scholars' Facsimiles & Reprints, Inc.,
P.O. Box 344, Delmar, New York 12054

© 1974 Scholars' Facsimiles & Reprints, Inc.,
All rights reserved

Printed in the United States of America

Library of Congress Cataloging in Publication Data

Combe, George, 1788-1858.
   The constitution of man considered in relation to external objects.

   Reprint of the 1834 ed. published by Allen and Ticknor, Boston.
   1. Psychology—Early works to 1850. 2. Man. I. Title.
BF111.C64   1974   150   74-16109
ISBN   0-8201-1136-8

Introduction

The early years of 19th-century Scotland were characterized by the struggle for power between the bleak doctrines of Calvinism and the ambiguous hopes of the emerging Unitarians. Published during the height of this controversy, the writings of George Combe offered a compelling alternative to these equally inadequate world views. Based on a phrenological model of the nature of man, Combe's philosophy gave to his confused and distressed countrymen their first sound reason for optimism, for Combe was able to offer an optimistic blueprint for social improvement, satisfying at once their penchant for organization and plan and their need to escape from an uncompromising Deity. Combe firmly believed that the phrenological discoveries of Gall and Spurzheim had revolutionized knowledge of the human mind equivalent to the advances of Copernicus and Newton in astronomy, and to him as their disciple was left the awesome task of saving humanity from itself through phrenology.

Phrenology was the brainchild of Franz Joseph Gall, a German physician whose interest in comparative anatomy had developed before earning his doctorate from the Vienna Medical School in 1788. His attention to brain anatomy and physiology was drawn from a childhood observation that those of his fellow students with good memories had large foreheads. His investigative research on this subject had been started at least by 1792. He attempted to correlate unusual personality traits in a given person with studies of his skull configuration and brain, examining the crania of his live patients, taking casts and collecting the skulls and brains after their deaths for extensive post-mortem examinations. His researches were sufficiently organized by 1796 to enable him to lecture on the subject. Two years later, he published his first phrenological article and by 1800 had attracted a student, Johann Christoph Spurzheim, to his side.

His lectures at Vienna created uneasiness among Church authorities and on 21 December, 1801 Emperor Francis issued a decree forbidding any further public demonstrations on the grounds that they led to materialism and therefore were anti-religious. Forced to leave Vienna in 1805 and accompanied by Spurzheim, Gall conducted a two-year tour through Germany, Switzerland, Holland, and Denmark. He lectured everywhere—frequently honored, often debated, and occasionally abused. Settling in Paris in 1807, he began his period of greatest productivity; although popular, he never received the scientific recognition he sought and remained a controversial figure until his death in 1828.

Gall's phrenological doctrine is best stated in his own words: "The object of all my researches is to found a doctrine on the function of the brain. The results of this doctrine ought to be the development of perfect knowledge of human nature. The possibility of any doctrine, in relation to the moral and intellectual function of the brain, supposes: 1. that moral and intellectual faculties are innate, 2. that their exercise or manifestations depend on organization, 3. that the brain is the organ of all the propensities, sentiments, and faculties, 4. that the brain is composed of as many particular organs as there are propensities, sentiments, and faculties which differ essentially from each other."[1] According to Gall's theory, there were twenty-seven such organs in man, nineteen of which he shared with the animal kingdom. In his studies based on comparative anatomy and physiology, he decided that the more fundamental faculties were located in the inferior and posterior portions of the brain. Most fundamental of all the faculties was the instinct to reproduce, followed in turn by love of offspring, friendship, and up to religion and firmness of character. He characterized the personality of each human being as dependent on the strength, balance and combination of these basic motivational forces located in the brain. His impact was such that Erwin Ackerknecht has called him "quite legitmately the godfather of the modern social sciences."[2]

But it was left to his student Spurzheim to popularize this new science, further developing Gall's original theories as he did so. These innovations led to his break with Gall in 1813. The following year Spurzheim initiated his first lecture tour, through England, Ireland and Scotland; his reception ranged from fair to very poor. During his three years in Great Britian and the following eight in Paris, Spurzheim wrote extensively on phrenology; an important work produced during this time concerned the application of phrenological principles to insanity.[3] There followed a second lecture tour in Great Britain, the success of which led to an invitation to speak in Boston, Massachusetts; he was widely acclaimed but died there suddenly of a fever in 1832.

The four primary changes Spurzheim initiated into the organology of Gall go beyond mere development and deserve to be classified more as innovations than explication. (1) Aiming for greater completeness, he increased the number of Gall's organs from 27 to 35; (2) Where Gall listed his faculties in an apparent biological and evolutionary order, Spurzheim rearranged them into a neat philosophical classification which followed the traditional division into [a.] feelings, or affective faculties and [b.] the intellectual faculties; (3) Within these new divisions he included certain qualities of the faculties which Gall would have considered as general attributes of all; (4) He disparaged Gall's pessimism by stating that there existed no evil faculties but only abuses of the normal ones. (For example, an excess of destructiveness corresponded to Gall's one of desire to murder, and an exaggerated acquisitiveness to his desire for theft.) This optimistic interpretation of human behavior was seized on by his followers in their fight to stress the importance of proper education to the health of the individual, and his role as representative of Christian excellence did much to ameliorate his detractors' accusations of materialism.

Present at one of Spurzheim's phrenology lectures at Edinburgh in 1816 was George Combe, an uninterested and disbelieving young lawyer. Born 21 October 1788, one of 17 children of an ill-educated but well-intentioned brewer, Combe had been reared in the strictest Calvinistic theology.[4] Illness often interrupted his education but after two years at the University of Edinburgh, he began a six-year apprenticeship in law and was admitted to the bar in 1810. Stoical and ambitious, Combe succeeded in his practice, but an entry in his diary for 1811 suggest his restlessness: "I have taken the imagination that I have powers of mind sufficient to write some useful book on human nature, and especially on the education and intellectual state of the middle ranks of society."[5]

By 1816 Combe was ripe for phrenology. In 1815, he had read Dr. John Gordon's scathing remarks on Gall and Spurzheim's first English work in the influential *Edinburgh Review*. The following year he accompanied a friend to a dissection and lecture in which Spurzheim demonstrated his method of unfolding the structures of the brain. He refuted Dr. Gordon's allegations point by point; Combe was convinced. He devoted increasing amounts of his leisure time to phrenological study and in the summer of 1817 went to Paris to study with Spurzheim. That year he published his first article for the *Scots Magazine*, following this with a series of defenses for phrenology in the *Literary and Statistical Magazine* in 1818, giving public lectures at Edinburgh the same year. His *Essays on Phrenology*, a revision of his periodical essays, appeared in 1819 and was well received. In February 1820 he helped found the first phrenological society, and in December 1823, began publication of the *Phrenological Journal* which ceased only with the death of his brother, Dr. Andrew Combe, in 1847. (After Andrew's death, George Combe wrote an extensive phrenological biography of his life. Included in it is a wealth of biographical information of his own childhood and adult life, with an account of how the brothers Combe viewed health and its maintenance through phrenological principles.)[6]

Up to this time, phrenological study had been biologically directed by the serious neuroanatomical research Gall performed with Spurzheim's assistance in their early collaboration.[7] It remained for Combe to follow Spurzheim's later direction, systematizing these studies for popular acceptance. Although he did not completely relinquish his legal practice until 1836, he spent increasing time and energy in lecturing and writing throughout the 1820s. During this decade phrenology gained a general acceptance in several countries, most notably in the United States; the publication of Combe's *Constitution of Man* in 1828, the year of Gall's death, helped to force the movement into the world's view.

In it, Combe discusses "the constitution, condition and prospects of Man." He disclaims any originality in thought, saying instead that he may have combined old facts in a new manner in his attempts to unite the scientific laws of nature with knowledge of man's constitution. His ultimate goal was a practical one: to acquire and use knowledge that will contribute to man's progress in his earthly life. He acknowledges God's involvement in that life but refuses to pursue it, stating that such study properly belongs in the theological sphere.

Despite his protestation, the modern reader can see the *Constitution* as a deeply religious book that provided him with a psychological and philosophical solution to his personal religious conflicts. Indoctrinated into the Calvinistic stress on the fall of man, he concluded early that he numbered among those fated for eternal damnation in hell. Confounded by the artificial religious fervor used by his country's leaders for their political expediency, distressed by the biogtry and hatred among the several religious sects, and confused by the security of seemingly-evil persons in their salvation (while he was tormented with the conviction of his damnation). He hoped for an end of doctrinal squabbles and sought instead a practical Christian spirit. His efforts in his phrenological writings were widely criticized as materialistic, deistic, antireligious, and even atheistic.[8]

Combe continued to publish and lecture; he engaged in a pamphlet duel with William Scott and lost his bid for the chair of logic at Edinburgh in 1836, defeated by Sir William Hamilton. Bitterly disappointed, he spent himself in travel on behalf of the phrenological cause. These travels brought him in September 1838 to America where he remained for twenty months, lecturing throughout the Northeast. Appropriately, he began his tour in the same hall in Boston where Spurzheim had introduced his phrenological concepts. His American audiences included many leaders in educational and reform movements, and he spoke privately with two presidents (Van Buren and Harrison). Throughout his stay, he kept a diary of his experiences; on his return to Scotland, he published his observations as *Notes on the United States of America*.[9] Their importance transcend the phrenological movement for their wealth of information on life in the United States, including detailed accounts of the weather, people, institutions, religion and slavery of his host country; he ends with a phrenological address to the people of America. Combe continued to travel throughout the remainder of his life, visiting all of the mid-European countries, returning several times to Germany.

His personal life was always secondary to the phrenological movement. In 1833, at forty-five years of age, Combe married Cecilia Siddons in what was apparently a successful but childless union. A sedate person, he dressed conservatively in somber colors until his marriage. And always emotionally controlled, he rarely smiled, and never cursed nor cried. Nevertheless, he was highly regarded by those close to him whom he repaid with deep loyalty and affection. As his health became more uncertain, his travels grew less frequent. He prepared work on his autobiography but increasing ill health forced him to dictate to his wife and ultimately prevented its completion when he died at a friend's water-cure establishment on 19 February 1858.

Combe's masterly *Constitution of Man* remains an important step in man's search for an understanding of his function in the world. In this work, Combe acknowledges his debt to Bishop Joseph Butler, best known for his *Analogy of Religion, Natural and Revealed, to the Constitution and Course of Nature* (1736). Butler preached a correlation between nature as a whole and human nature specifically which operates according to certain laws. According to how man deals with these laws, his life is either one of pain and misery or pleasure and happiness. Through reflection, man can perceive the consequences of his actions. Combe adapts this idea in the text of his work. His laws are threefold: the physical laws of the inorganic world, those of living creatures, and the moral laws of man and his society. By the 1820s these first two postulates had gained a general acceptance, but Combe's third postulate, his suggestion that there existed moral laws that acted on man's behavior, appeared to many to impinge on God's dominion. But supported by the ideas of the famed Cambridge geologist, Adam Sedgwick, Combe continued to prove the depths of human nature.[10]

Essential to an understanding of this human nature was a preliminary philosophy of mind. A product of the latter part of the Scottish enlightenment, Combe had received the standard exposure to Scottish thinkers: Francis Hutcheson, Thomas Reid, Adam Smith, Dugald Stewart, and Thomas Brown. These philosophers had accustomed him to a faculty psychology but as he focused on the live, functioning human body in a material world, Combe needed a psychology related to the body but clear and specific enough for study and comprehension. He found this in phrenology, specifically in Spurzheim's writings. Combe largely used Spurzheim's thirty-five faculties in their arrangement of functional purpose but it was his teacher's manuscript copy of *A Sketch of the Natural Laws of Man* (published 1825) that served as the catalyst for Combe.

In his attempts to understand man and his nature, Combe ranged from discussions of comparative psychology to that of the role of heredity, both individually and racially. He received the germ of his ideas on heredity from a contemporary British anthropologist and psychiatrist, Dr. J.C. Prichard (*Researches into the Physical History of Mankind*, 1826). Combe added his belief in God's creation of most of man's mental faculties to relate to objects in the external world (thereby developing a kind of object-relations psychology). But as these faculties strongly tended to seek their own individual ends, the remaining faculties need knowledge and wisdom to organize and coordinate their activities toward progressive ends. Only these higher moral and intellectual capacities of man can learn "that the rewards and punishments of human actions are infinitely more complete, certain and efficacious, in this life, than is generally believed." In other words, the individual man does play an active role in the progress and shaping of himself and his world, and is not immediately subject to the will of a Supreme Being.[11] Combe urged man to use his new knowledge for social design, as "man must live in society to be either virtuous, useful, or happy; that the social atmosphere is to the mind what air is to the lungs; that while an individual cannot exist to virtuous ends out of society, he cannot exist in a right frame in it, if the moral atmosphere with which he is surrounded be deeply contaminated with vice and error."

An air of optimism permeates the *Constitution* reminiscent of the Enlightenment. Cojoined is another 18th-century concept, that of nature and man's place therein. In the "great chain of being," man is at the top in the real world which was not only made for man but gradually improved by God to prepare it for man's inhabitance.[12] At the same time, man appears to be adapted to this world already adapted for him. He is anomalous for Combe—on the one hand he is made in God's image, on the other his behavior often resembles that of the lowest orders, even to existing at their relatively simple level taking pleasure from the basic physiological life processes. But this denies the higher side of man given by God, his "moral sentiments and reflecting faculties." It is through their use that man has acquired knowledge about his world and how best to adapt to it. Both man and knowledge are progressive. The pace is accelerating; phrenology and, for that matter, Combe's book (for all his modest disavowal) makes possible a marked increase in tempo. This progressive view of the world also meant that as man came to see more of God's plan for all time, he would need to accept both his behavior and his religion to fit this new knowledge. This destroyed the old, secure hierarchy of the "saved" and the "damned" with which the Presbyterians had comforted themselves against the stagnation of their sociological development. Although man could become perfect only through God, he was entirely capable of self-motivated progress toward perfection through his understanding of God's plan. This goal fitted well with the hope for reform of the day that was at least partly realized in the passage in Great Britain of the Reform Bill of 1832. Largely based on Bentham's principle of the "greatest good for the greatest number," this echoes the credo of Combe's life efforts.

The *Constitution of Man* fulfilled its author's hope for popular dissemination. His first edition of 1,500 copies omitted his deliberations on moral responsibility and on the psychology of animals in an attempt to avoid the excessive controversy they provoked. Controversy still greeted the book, but it sold steadily. A bequest in 1832 from William R. Henderson made possible the sale of a number of the books at reduced prices and stimulated Combe to prepare his second, revised edition in 1833. A special "People's Edition" printed in double column sold nearly 60,000 copies in the course of the next four years. An American edition was published as early as 1829 and translations gradually appeared in French, German, Italian, Polish, Spanish, and Swedish. Perhaps the ultimate step in its widespread use for popular education was its republication in raised type for those with visual impairment, by Dr. Samuel Gridley Howe.[13] About mid-century, it was estimated that more than 300,000 copies had been sold. It has been considered one of the most popular books of the 19th century, so popular that it has been described as the only book to join the Bible and *Pilgrim's Progress* on the shelf in the home of the common man.

In addition to his enormous phrenological impact, Combe both directly and indirectly influenced many leading minds of the 19th century in the broad and growing areas of education and the growth of social sciences. Horace Mann completely adopted his philosophy of education and had the *Constitution of Man* issued as a text in the Massachusetts school system. Phrenology was one of the great intellectual movements of the century, and as Robert N. Young has so well indicated, it occupied a similar if less scientifically successful position as did evolution later in the century.[14] Because George Combe seriously attempted to understand man and his individual and social behavior, he has achieved a secure if minor position in the history of the social sciences.

Eric T. Carlson, M.D.

New York, New York

The author wishes to acknowledge the assistance of Beatrice T. Heveran and the support in part on N.I.H. grant LM 00910 from the National Library of Medicine.

1. Franz J. Gall, *On the Functions of the Brain and of Each of Its Parts*, 6 vols. (Boston: Marsh, Capen and Lyon, 1835), 1:55.

2. Erwin H. Ackerknecht and Henri V. Vallois, *Franz Joseph Gall, Inventor of Phrenology and His Collection* (Madison, Wis.: University of Wisconsin Medical School, 1956), p. 36.

3. Johann C. Spurzheim, *Observations on the Deranged Manifestations of the Mind, or Insanity*. (London: Baldwin, Cradock and Joy, 1817; reprinted by Scholars' Facsimiles & Reprints in 1970). Andrew Combe wrote the only other phrenological work on insanity *(Observations on Mental Derangement*, Edinburgh: John Anderson, 1831; first American edition, 1834, reprinted by Scholars' Facsimiles & Reprints in 1972). For the general impact of phrenology on psychiatry, see Eric T. Carlson, "The Influence of Phrenology on Early American Psychiatric Thought," *American Journal of Psychiatry*, 115 (1958): 535-38.

4. Charles Gibbon, *The Life of George Combe*, 2 vols. (London: Macmillan and Co., 1878).

5. Ibid., 1:73.

6. George Combe, *The Life and Correspondence of Andrew Combe, M.D.* (Edinburgh: Mac Lachlan and Stewart, 1850).

7. Edwin Clarke and C.D. O'Malley, *The Human Brain and Spinal Cord* (Berkeley: University of California Press, 1968).

8. Anthony A. Walsh, "George Combe: A Portrait of a Heretofore Generally Unknown Behaviorist," *Journal of the History of the Behavioral Sciences* 7 (1971): 269-78.

9. George Combe *Notes on the United States of North America*, 2 vols. (Philadelphia: Carey and Hart, 1841).

10. Charles C. Gillespie, *Genesis and Geology* (Cambridge: Harvard University Press, 1951).

11. Cameron A. Grant, "Combe on Phrenology and Free Will: A Note on XIXth Century Secularism," *Journal of the History of Ideas* 26 (1965): 141-47.

12. Arthur O. Lovejoy, *The Great Chain of Being* (New York: Harper and Brothers, 1960).

13. John D. Davies, *Phrenology, Fad and Science* (New Haven: Yale University Press, 1955).

14. Robert M. Young, *Mind, Brain and Adaptation in the Nineteenth Century* (Oxford: Clarendon Press, 1970).

THE

CONSTITUTION OF MAN

CONSIDERED IN

RELATION TO EXTERNAL OBJECTS.

BY

GEORGE COMBE.

Vain is the ridicule with which one sees some persons will divert themselves, upon finding lesser pains considered as instances of divine punishment. There is no possibility of answering or evading the general thing here intended, without denying all final causes.—*Butler's Analogy.*

———

THIRD AMERICAN EDITION.

———

BOSTON:
ALLEN AND TICKNOR.
1834.

Charles A. Green, Printer, 19 Water-street.

PREFACE TO THE AMERICAN EDITION.

The author of the following work is known in this country by his Essays on Phrenology. Few men in Great Britain have discovered more sincere devotion to this subject itself, or more zeal in communicating it to others, than Mr. Combe. He shows every where in what he has written on phrenology a full conviction that his favourite science is founded in nature; that it will aid the study and progress of intellectual philosophy; that for want of its aids this philosophy has hitherto necessarily been imperfect; that, in short, phrenology is susceptible of a wide and useful application, and is destined to exert an important influence over the whole circle of human interests.

The following essay on the Constitution of Man is founded on phrenology; at least, the phrenological classification of the human faculties is adopted by the writer as the basis of his observations. This can hardly be objected to. To those who have studied phrenology it will be a recommendation; and to those who know it only by name, sufficient is brought into view in the volume to give them a general notion of a science which has engaged many able minds, and which in its measure belongs to the intellectual labours of the age. Mr. Combe does not appear to use it, in order to make converts to the phrenological faith; but rather brings it in to promote the great object of his present publication. This object is human happiness in an extended use of the term. He says, in amount, to lessen misery and increase happiness is his great purpose, and to accomplish this, his labour has been to discover as many of the contrivances of the Creator, for effecting beneficial purposes as possible; and secondly, to point out in what manner by accommodating our conduct to these contrivances we may attain one great end of our being.

In prosecution of this design, Mr. Combe's first inquiries are directed to the external world. He regards things first, as they are; and secondly, the purposes of their creation. These inquiries involve many very interesting views relating to the world without us; the actual condition of things; their mutual influences, whether remote or near; whether contingent or necessary. The circumstances under which phenomena take place, or with the author, the established and constant modes or processes according to which phenomena are produced, are *laws*, rules of action; and the first part of his work treats of *natural laws*. In the second chapter, Mr. Combe treats of the constitution of man, and its relations to external things. In the first place man is regarded as a *physical* being, composed of physical elements, and to a certain extent, and under like circumstances, exhibiting like phenomena with the objects of the external material world. In the next place he is viewed as an *organized* being, and the laws of his organization, together with the correspondences and differences between these and the natural laws are pointed out. The moral and intellectual constitution of man are treated under precisely similar aspects. The whole subject is developed with great skill, and made clear and interesting by a great variety of very happy illustrations.

The main design of this work is never lost sight of. This is to make men happier and better,—to show how the human race may be as happy as the constitution of man actually fits it to be. To do this, the author assumes that this constitution was designed to harmonize perfectly with itself in all its parts; and also with the whole creation so far as it is capable of being brought into relations with it. In the next place he labours to show that in order to the accomplishment of this design, sufficiently varied and active powers have been committed to man, and if he fail of the happiness for which he was designed here, it is not because he wants capacity of felicity, but because he has misused the powers with which he has been blessed. Human happiness then consists in an exact accordance of all the laws which are in operation within us, and again of these with all the laws which govern the external world. Human misery is the direct and necessary consequence of an infringement of these laws, or of some of them. The same skill is shown in treating this part of the work which has been noticed as characterizing the other. The same felicity of illustration is every where discoverable. The earnestness of truth is the prevailing characteristic, and a truly benevolent purpose marks every page.

Mr. Combe's work should be placed with those, of which so many within a few years have appeared, which are devoted to the all-absorbing topic of *Education*. It treats of moral, intellectual, and physical education. This is not formally done under so many distinct heads. But the whole course of reasoning of the author, and the whole array of all his illustrations, have it always obviously in view to show how the highest cultivation of each of these may be most surely brought about.

The publishers have printed this edition from a belief that there is much in the work to interest the community. It has novelty to reward the general inquirer, and it presents the well known under novel aspects. There is one class amongst us who may study it with much advantage. Scholars are referred to, a class here too small to form a distinct order with habits of their own, and who insensibly fall into those which although not mischievous to the multitude on the score of health, too often make ill health the portion of the sedentary student, and bring upon him premature decay. To all classes it is recommended, and the various learning, and acuteness of the author well fit him to write a book which addresses its instructions to the whole community.

PREFACE.

This Essay would not have been presented to the public, had I not believed that it contains views of the constitution, condition, and prospects of Man, which deserve attention ; but these, I trust, are not ushered forth with anything approaching to a presumptuous spirit. I lay no claim to originality of conception. My first notions of the natural laws were derived from an unpublished manuscript of Dr. SPURZHEIM, with the perusal of which I was honoured some years ago ; and all my inquiries and meditations since have impressed me more and more with a conviction of their importance. The materials employed lie open to all. Taken separately, I would hardly say that a new truth has been presented in the following work. The parts have all been admitted and employed again and again, by writers on morals, from SOCRATES down to the present day. In this respect, there is nothing new under the sun. The only novelty in this Essay respects the relations which acknowledged truths hold to each other. Physical laws of nature, affecting our physical condition, as well as regulating the whole material system of the universe, are universally acknowledged, and constitute the elements of natural philosophy and chemical science. Physiologists, medical practitioners, and all who take medical aid, admit the existence of *organic laws ;* and the science of government, legislation, education, indeed our whole train of conduct through life, proceed upon the admission of laws in morals. Accordingly, the laws of nature have formed an interesting subject of inquiry to philosophers of all ages ; but, so far as I am aware, no author has hitherto attempted to point out, in a combined and systematic form, the relations between these laws and the constitution of Man ; which must, nevertheless, be done, before our knowledge of them can be beneficially applied. The great object of the following Essay is to exhibit these relations, with a view to the improvement of education, and the regulation of individual conduct.

But, although my purpose is practical, a theory of Mind forms an essential element in the execution of the plan. Without it, no comparison can be instituted between the natural constitution of man and external objects. Phrenology appears to me to be the clearest, most complete, and best supported system of Human Nature, which has hitherto been taught ; and I have assumed it as the basis of this Essay. But the practical value of the views now to be unfolded does not depend on Phrenology. This theory of Mind itself is valuable, only in so far as it is *a just exposition* of what previously existed in human nature. We are physical, organic, and moral beings, acting under the sanction of general laws, let the merits of Phrenology be what they may. Individuals will, under the impulse of passion, or by the direction of intellect, hope, fear, wonder, perceive, and act, whether the degree in which they habitually do so, be ascertainable on phrenological principles or not. In so far, therefore, as this Essay treats of the known qualities of Man, it may be instructive even to those who contemn Phrenology as unfounded ; while it can prove useful to no one, if it shall depart from the true elements of mental philosophy, by whatever system these may be expounded.

I have endeavoured to avoid all religious controversy. 'The object of Moral Philosophy,' says Mr. STEWART, 'is to ascertain the general rules of a wise and virtuous conduct in life, in so far as these rules may be discovered by the unassisted light of nature; that is, by an examination of the principles of the human constitution, and of the circumstances in which Man is placed.'* By following this method of inquiry, Dr. HUTCHESON, Dr. ADAM SMITH, Dr. REID, Mr. STEWART, and Dr. THOMAS BROWN, have, in succession, produced highly interesting and instructive works on Moral Science; and the present Essay is an humble attempt to pursue the same plan, with the aid of the new lights afforded by Phrenology.

Edinburgh, 9th June, 1828.

---

* Outlines of Moral Philosophy, p. 1.

CONTENTS.

CHAPTER I.

On Natural Laws, ... 1

CHAPTER II.

Of the Constitution of Man, and its Relations to External Objects, ... 16
Section I. Man considered as a Physical Being, . . 17
    II. Man considered as an Organized Being, . . 20
    III. Man considered as an Animal—Moral—and Intellectual Being, ... 24
    IV. The Faculties of Man compared with each other; or the supremacy of the Moral Sentiments and Intellect, ... 28
    V. The Faculties of Man compared with External Objects, ... 46
    VI. On the sources of Human Happiness, and the conditions requisite for maintaining it, . . 52
    VII. Application of the Natural Laws to the practical arrangements of Life, ... 65

CHAPTER III.

To what extent are the Miseries of Mankind referable to Infringements of the Laws of Nature, . . 71
Section I. Calamities arising from infringements of the Physical Laws, ... 71
    II. On the Evils that befall Mankind, from infringement of the Organic Laws, . . . - 76
    III. Calamities arising from infringement of the Moral Law, ... 141
    IV. Moral advantages of Punishment, . . . 178

CHAPTER IV.

On the combined operation of the Natural Laws, . 181
Conclusion, ... 197

APPENDIX.

Note I. Natural Laws, [Text, p. 1.] 207
    II. Organic Laws, [Text, p. 76.] 211
    III. Death, Decreasing Mortality, [Text, p. 128.] . 215
    IV. Moral Law, [Text, p. 159.] 219

ESSAY

ON THE

CONSTITUTION OF MAN,

AND ITS RELATIONS TO EXTERNAL OBJECTS.

CHAPTER I.

ON NATURAL LAWS.

A STATEMENT of the evidence of a great intelligent First Cause is given in the 'Phrenological Journal,' and in the 'System of Phrenology.' I hold this existence as capable of demonstration. By NATURE, I mean the workmanship of this great Being, such as it is revealed to our minds by our senses and faculties.

In natural science, three subjects of inquiry may be distinguished. 1st. What exists? 2dly. What is the purpose or design of what exists; and, 3dly. Why was what exists designed for such uses as it evidently subserves? For example,—It is matter of fact that arctic regions and torrid zones exist,—that a certain kind of moss is most abundant in Lapland in mid-winter,—that the rein-deer feeds on it, and enjoys high health and vigour in situations where most other animals would die; further, it is matter of fact that camels exist in Africa,—that they have broad hooves, and stomachs fitted to retain water for a length of time, and that they flourish amid arid tracts of sand, where the rein-deer would not live for a day. All this falls under the enquiry, What exists? But in contemplating the foregoing facts, it is impossible not to infer that one object of the Lapland moss is to feed the rein-deer, and one purpose of the deer is to assist man : and that, in like manner, broad feet have been given to the camel to enable it to walk on sand; and a retentive stomach to fit it for arid places in which water is not found except at wide intervals. These are enquiries into the use or purpose of what exists. In like manner, we may enquire, What purpose do sandy deserts and desolate heaths subserve in the economy of nature? In short, an enquiry into the use or purpose of any object that exists, *is merely an examination of its relations to other objects and beings, and of the modes in which it affects them;* and this is quite a legitimate exercise of the human intellect. But, 3dly. we may ask, why were the physical elements of nature created such as they are? Why were summer, autumn, spring, and winter introduced? Why were animals formed of organized matter? These are inquiries why what exists was made such as it is, or into the will of the Deity in creation. Now, man's perceptive faculties are adequate to the first inquiry, and his reflective faculties to the second; but it may well be doubted whether he has powers suited to the third. My investigations are confined to the first and second, and I do not discuss the third.

A *law*, in the common acceptation, denotes a rule of action; its existence indicates an established and constant mode, or process, according to which phenomena take place; and this is the sense in which I shall use it, when treating of physical substances and beings. For example, water and heat are substances; and water presents different appearances, and manifests certain qualities, according to the altitude of its situation, and the degree of heat with which it is combined. When at the level of the sea, and combined with that portion of heat indicated by 32° of Fahrenheit's thermometer, it freezes or becomes solid; when combined with the portion denoted by 212° of that instrument, it rises into vapour or steam. Here, water and heat are the substances,—the freezing and rising in vapour are the appearances or phenomena presented by them; and when we say that these take place according to a Law of Nature, we mean only that these modes of action appear, to our intellects, to be established in the very constitution of the water and heat, and in their natural relationship to each other; and that the processes of freezing and rising in vapour are their constant appearances, when combined in these proportions, other conditions being the same.

The ideas chiefly to be kept in view are, 1st. That all substances and beings have received a definite natural constitution; 2dly. That every mode of action, which is said to take place according to a natural law, is inherent in the constitution of the substance, or being, that acts; and, 3dly, That the mode of action described is universal and invarible, wherever and whenever the substances, or beings, are found in the same condition. For example, water, at the level of the sea, freezes and boils, at the same temperature, in China and in France, in Peru and in England; and there is no exception to the regularity with which it exhibits these appearances, when all its conditions are the same: For *cæteris paribus* is a condition which pervades all departments of science, phrenology included. If water be carried to the top of a mountain 20,000 feet high, it boils at a lower temperature than 212°, but this again depends on its relationship to the air, and takes place also according to fixed and invariable principles. The air exerts a great pressure on the water. At the level of the sea the pressure is nearly the same in all quarters of the globe, and in that situation the freezing points and boiling points correspond all over the world; but on the top of a high mountain the pressure is much less, and the vapour not being held down by so great a power of resistance, rises at a lower degree of heat than 212°. But this change of appearances does not indicate a change in the constitution of the water and the heat, but only a variation of the circumstances in which they are placed; and hence it is not correct to say, that water boiling on the tops of high mountains, at a lower temperature than 212°, is an exception to the general law of nature: there never are exceptions to the laws of nature; for the Creator is too wise and too powerful to make imperfect or inconsistent arrangements. The error is in the human mind inferring the law to be, that water boils at 212° in all altitudes; when the real law is only that it boils at that temperature, *at the level of the sea*, in all countries; and that it boils at a lower temperature, the higher it is carried, because there the pressure of the atmosphere is diminished.

Intelligent beings exist, and are capable of modifying their actions. By means of their faculties, the laws impressed by the Creator on physical substances become known to them; and, when perceived, constitute laws to them, by which to regulate their conduct. For example, it is a physical law, that boiling water destroys the muscular and nervous systems of man. This is the result purely of the constitution of the body, and the relation between it and heat; and man cannot alter or suspend that law. But whenever the human intellect perceives the relation, and the consequences of violating it, the mind is prompted to avoid infringement, in order to shun the torture attached by the Creator to the decomposition of the human body by heat.

Similar views have long been taught by philosophers and divines. Bishop BUTLER, in particular, says:—'An Author of Nature being supposed, it is not so much a deduction of reason as a matter of experience, that we are thus under his government, in the same sense as we are under the government of civil magistrates. Because the annexing pleasure to some actions, and pain to others, in our power to do or forbear, and giving notice of this appointment beforehand to those whom it concerns, *is the proper formal notion of government*. Whether the pleasure or pain which thus follows upon our behaviour, be owing to the Author of Nature's acting upon us every moment which we feel it, or to his having at once contrived and executed his own part in the plan of the world, makes no alteration as to the matter before us. For, if civil magistrates could make the sanctions of their laws take place, without interposing at all, after they had passed them, without a trial, and the formalities of an execution; if they were able to make their laws execute themselves, or every offender to execute them upon himself, we should be just in the same sense under their government then as we are now; but in a much higher degree and more perfect manner. *Vain is the ridicule with which one sees some persons will divert themselves, upon finding* LESSER PAINS CONSIDERED AS INSTANCES OF DIVINE PUNISHMENT. THERE IS NO POSSIBILITY OF ANSWERING OR EVADING *the general thing here intended*, WITHOUT DENYING ALL FINAL CAUSES. For, final causes being admitted, the pleasures and pains now mentioned must be admitted too, as instances of them. And if they are, if GOD annexes delight to some actions, with an apparent design to induce us to act so and so, then he not only dispenses happiness and misery, but also rewards and punishes actions. If, for example, the *pain which we feel upon doing what tends to the destruction of our bodies*, suppose upon too near approaches to fire, or upon wounding ourselves, be *appointed by the Author of Nature to prevent our doing what thus tends to our destruction;* this is ALTOGETHER AS MUCH AN INSTANCE OF HIS PUNISHING OUR ACTIONS, and consequently of our being under his government, as declaring, by a voice from Heaven, that, if we acted so, He would inflict such pain upon us, and inflict it whether it be greater or less.'[*]

If, then, the reader keep in view that GOD is the creator; that Nature, in the general sense, means the world which He has made; and, in a more limited sense, the particular

---

[*] BUTLER's Works, vol. i. p. 44. Similar observations by other authors will be found in the Appendix, No 1.

constitution which he has bestowed on any special object, of which we may be treating, and that a Law of Nature means the established mode in which that constitution acts, and the obligation thereby imposed on intelligent beings to attend to it, he will be in no danger of misunderstanding my meaning.

Every natural object has received a definite constitution, in virtue of which it acts in a particular way. There must, therefore, be as many natural laws, as there are distinct modes of action of substances and beings, viewed by themselves. But substances and beings stand in certain relations to each other, and modify each other's action in an established and definite manner, according to that relationship; altitude, for instance, modifies the effect of heat upon water. There must, therefore, be also as many laws of nature, as there are *relations* between different substances and beings.

It is impossible, in the present state of knowledge, to elucidate all these laws: countless years may elapse before they shall be discovered; but we may investigate some of the most familiar and striking of them. Those that most readily present themselves bear reference to the great classes into which the objects around us may be divided, namely, Physical, Organic, and Intelligent. I shall therefore confine myself to the physical laws, the organic laws, and the laws which characterise intelligent beings.

1st. The Physical Laws embrace all the phenomena of mere matter; a heavy body, for instance, when unsupported, falls to the ground with a certain accelerating force, in proportion to the distance which it falls, and its own density; and this motion is said to take place according to the law of gravitation. An acid applied to a vegetable blue colour, converts it into red, and this is said to take place according to a chemical law.

2dly. Organised substances and beings stand higher in the scale of creation, and have properties peculiar to themselves. They act, and are acted upon, in conformity with their constitution, and are therefore said to be subject to a peculiar set of laws, termed the Organic. The distinguishing characteristic of this class of objects, is, that the individuals of them derive their existence from other organized beings, are nourished by food, and go through a regular process of growth and decay. Vegetables and Animals are the two great subdivisions of it. The organic laws are different from the merely physical. A stone, for example, does not spring from a parent stone; it does not take food from its parent, the earth, or air; it does not increase in vigour for a time, and then decay and suffer dissolution, all which processes characterise vegetables and animals. The organic laws are superior to the merely physical. For example, a living man, or animal, may be placed in an oven, along with the carcass of a dead animal, and remain exposed to a heat, which will completely bake the dead flesh, and yet come out alive, and not seriously injured. The dead flesh is mere physical matter, and its decomposition by the heat instantly commences; but the living animal is able, by its organic qualities, to counteract and resist to a certain extent, that influence. The expression Organic Laws, therefore, indicates that every phenomenon connected with the production, health, growth, decay, and death of vegetables and animals, takes place with undeviating regularity, whenever circumstances are the same. Animals are the chief objects of my present observations.

3dly. Intelligent beings stand still higher in the scale than merely organised matter, and embrace all animals that have distinct consciousness, from the lowest of the inferior creatures up to man. The great divisions of this class are into Intelligent and Animal—and into Intelligent and Moral creatures. The dog, horse, and elephant, for instance, belong to the first class, because they possess some degree of intelligence, and certain animal propensities, but no moral feelings; man belongs to the second, because he possesses all the three. These various faculties have received a definite constitution from the Creator, and stand in determinate relationship to external objects: for example, a healthy palate cannot feel wormwood sweet, nor sugar bitter: a healthy eye cannot see a rod partly plunged in water straight, because the water so modifies the rays of light, as to give to the stick the appearance of being crooked; a healthy Benevolence cannot feel gratified with murder, nor a healthy Conscientiousness with fraud. As, therefore, the mental faculties have received a precise constitution, have been placed in fixed and definite relations to external objects, and act regularly, we speak of their acting according to rules or laws, and call these the Moral and Intellectual Laws.

In short, the expression 'laws of nature,' when properly used, signifies the rules of action impressed on objects and beings by their natural constitution. Thus, when we say, that by the physical law, a ship sinks when a plank starts from her side, we mean, that, by the constitution of the ship, and the water, and the relation subsisting between them, the ship sinks when the plank starts.

Several important principles strike us very early in attending to the natural laws, viz. 1st. Their independence of each other; 2dly. Obedience to each of them is attended with its own reward, and disobedience with its own punishment; 3dly. They are universal, unbending, and invariable in their operation; 4thly. They are in harmony with the constitution of man.

1. The independence of the natural laws may be illustrated thus;—A ship floats because a part of it being immersed, displaces a weight of water equal to its whole weight, leaving the remaining part above the fluid. A ship, therefore, will float on the surface of the water as long as these physical conditions are observed; no matter although the men in it should infringe other natural laws;

as, for example, although they should rob, murder, blaspheme, and commit every species of debauchery; and it will sink whenever the physical conditions are subverted, however strictly the crew and passengers may obey the other laws here adverted to. In like manner, a man who swallows poison, which destroys the stomach or intestines, will die, just because an organic law has been infringed, and because it is independent of others, although the man should have taken the drug by mistake, or been the most pious and charitable individual on earth. Or, thirdly, a man may cheat, lie, steal, tyrannise, and in short break a great variety of the moral laws, and nevertheless be fat and rubicund, if he sedulously observed the organic laws of temperance and exercise, which determine the condition of the body; while, on the other hand, an individual who neglects these, may pine in disease, and be racked with torturing pains, although at the very moment, he may be devoting his mind to the highest duties of humanity.

2. Obedience to each law is attended with its own reward, and disobedience with its own punishment. Thus the mariners who preserve their ship in accordance with the physical laws, reap the reward of sailing in safety; and those who permit its departure from them, are punished by the ship sinking. Those who obey the moral law, enjoy the intense internal delights that spring from active moral faculties; they render themselves, moreover, objects of affection and esteem to moral and intelligent beings, who, in consequence, confer on them many other gratifications. Those who disobey that law, are tormented with insatiable desires, which, from the nature of things, cannot be gratified; they are punished by the perpetual craving of whatever portion of moral sentiment they possess, for higher enjoyments, which are never attained; and they are objects of dislike and malevolence to other beings in the same condition as themselves, who inflict on them the evils dictated by their own provoked propensities. Those who

obey the organic laws, reap the reward of health and vigour of body and buoyancy of mind ; those who break them are punished by sickness, feebleness, and languor.

3. The natural laws are universal, invariable, and unbending. When the physical laws are subverted in China or Kamschatka, there is no instance of a ship floating there more than in England; and, when they are observed, there is no instance of a vessel sinking in any one of these countries more than in another. There is no example of men, in any country, enjoying the mild and generous internal joys, and the outward esteem and love that attend obedience to the moral law, while they give themselves up to the dominion of brutal propensities. There is no example, in any latitude or longitude, or in any age, of men who entered life with a constitution in perfect harmony with the organic laws, and who continued to obey these laws throughout, being, in consequence of this obedience, visited with pain and disease; and there are no instances of men who were born with constitutions at variance with the organic laws, and who lived in habitual disobedience to them, enjoying that sound health and vigour of body, that are the rewards of obedience.

4. The natural laws are in harmony with the whole constitution of man, the moral and intellectual powers being supreme. For example, if ships had sunk when they were in accordance with the physical law, this would have outraged the perceptions of Causality, and offended Benevolence and Justice; but as they float, the physical is, in this instance, in harmony with the moral and intellectual law. If men who rioted in drunkenness and debauchery, had thereby established health and increased their happiness, this, again, would have been in discord with our intellectual and moral perceptions; but the opposite result is in harmony with them.

It will be subsequently shown, that our moral sentiments desire universal happiness. If the physical and organic laws are constituted in harmony with them, it ought to follow that the natural laws, when obeyed, conduce to the happiness of moral and intelligent beings, who are called on to observe them; and that the evil consequences or punishments resulting from disobedience, are calculated to enforce stricter attention and obedience to the laws, that these beings may escape from the miseries of infringement, and return to the advantages of observance. For example, according to this view, when a ship sinks, in consequence of a plank starting, the punishment ought to impress upon the spectators the absolute necessity of having every plank secure and strong, before going to sea again, a condition indispensable to their safety. When sickness and pain follow a debauche, they serve to urge a more scrupulous obedience to the organic laws, that the individual may escape death, which is the inevitable consequence of too great and continued disobedience to these laws, and enjoy health, which is the reward of opposite conduct. When discontent, irritation, hatred, and other mental annoyances, arise out of infringement of the moral law, this punishment is calculated to induce the offender to return to obedience, that he may enjoy the rewards attached to it.

When the transgression of any natural law is excessive, and so great that return to obedience is impossible, one purpose of death, which then ensues, may be to deliver the individual from a continuation of the punishment which could then do him no good. Thus, when, from infringement of a physical law, a ship sinks at sea, and leaves men immersed in water, without the possibility of reaching land, their continued existence in that state would be one of cruel and protracted suffering; and it is advantageous to them to have their mortal life extinguished at once by drowning, thereby withdrawing them from further agony. In like manner, if a man in the vigour of life, so far infringe any organic law as to destroy the function of a vital organ, the heart, for instance, or the lungs, or the brain, it is better for him to have his life cut short, and his pain put an end to, than to have it protracted under all the tortures of an organic existence without lungs, without a heart, or without a brain, if such a state were possible, which, for this wise reason, it is not.

I do not intend to predicate anything concerning the perfectibility of man by obedience to the laws of nature. The system of sublunary creation, so far as we perceive it, does not appear to be one of optimism; yet benevolent design, in its constitution, is undeniable. PALEY says, 'Nothing remains but the first supposition, that GOD, when he created the human species, wished them happiness, and made for them the provisions which he has made, with that view and for that purpose. The same argument may be proposed in different terms: Contrivance proves design; and the predominant tendency of the contrivance indicates the disposition of the designer. The world *abounds with contrivances;* and ALL THE CONTRIVANCES *which we are acquainted with, are directed to beneficial purposes.*' —PALEY's Mor. Phil. Edinb. 1816, p. 51. My object is to discover as many of the contrivances of the Creator, for effecting beneficial purposes, as possible; and to point out in what manner, by accommodating our conduct to these contrivances, we may lessen our misery and increase our happiness.

I do not intend to teach that the natural laws, discernible by unassisted reason, are sufficient for the *salvation* of man without revelation. Human interests regard this world and the next. To enjoy this world, I humbly maintain, that man must discover and obey the natural laws; for example, to ensure health to offspring, the parents must be healthy, and the children after birth must be treated in conformity to the organic laws; to fit them for usefulness in society, they must be instructed in their own constitution, —in that of external objects and beings, and taught to act rationally in reference to these. Revelation does not communicate complete or scientific information concerning the best mode of pursuing even our legitimate temporal interests, probably because faculties have been given to man to discover arts, sciences, and the natural laws, and to adapt his conduct to them. The physical, moral, and intellectual nature of man, is itself open to investigation by our natural faculties ; and numerous practical duties resulting from our constitution are discoverable, which are not treated of in detail in the inspired volume ; the mode of preserving health, for example ; of pursuing with success a temporal calling ; of discovering the qualities of men with whom we mean to associate our interests ; and many others. My object, I repeat, is to investigate the natural constitution of the human body and mind, their relations to external objects and beings in this world, and the courses of action that, in consequence, appear to be beneficial or hurtful.

Man's spiritual interests belong to the sphere of revelation ; and I distinctly declare, that I do not teach, that obedience to the natural laws is sufficient for salvation in a future state. Revelation prescribes certain requisites for salvation, which may be divided into two classes ; first, faith or belief: and, secondly, the performance of certain practical duties, not as meritorious of salvation, but as the native result of that faith, and the necessary evidence of its sincerity. The natural laws form no guide as to faith; but so far as I can perceive, their dictates and those of revelation coincide in all matters relating to practical duties in temporal affairs.

It may be asked, whether mere *knowledge* of the natural laws is sufficient to insure observance of them ? Certainly not. Mere knowledge of music does not enable one to play on an instrument, nor of anatomy to perform skilfully a surgical operation. Practical training, and the aid of every motive that can interest the feelings, are necessary to lead individuals to obey the natural laws. Religion, in particular, may furnish motives highly conducive to this obedience. But, it must never be forgotten, that although mere knowledge is not all-sufficient, it is a primary and indispensable requisite to regular observance; and that it is as impossible, effectually and systematically to obey the natural laws without knowing them, as it is to infringe them with impunity, although from ignorance of their existence. Some persons are of opinion that Christianity alone suffices, not only for man's salvation, which I do not dispute, but for his guidance in all practical virtues, without knowledge of, or obedience to, the laws of nature; but from this notion I respectfully dissent. It appears to me, that one reason why vice and misery, in this world, do not diminish in proportion to preaching, is, because the natural laws are too much overlooked, and very rarely considered as having any relation to practical conduct.

Connected with this subject, it is proper to state, that I do not maintain that the world is arranged on the principle of Benevolence exclusively: my idea is, that it is constituted in harmony with the whole faculties of man; the moral sentiments and intellect holding the supremacy. What is meant by creation being constituted in harmony with the whole faculties of man, is this. Suppose that we should see two men holding a third in a chair, and a fourth drawing a tooth from his head:—While we contemplated this bare act, and knew nothing of the intention with which it was done, and of the consequences that would follow, we would set it down as purely cruel; and say, that, although it might be in harmony with Destructiveness, it could not be so with Benevolence. But, when we were told that the individual in the chair was a patient, the operator a dentist, the two men his assistants, and that the object of all the parties was to deliver the first from violent torture, we would then perceive that Destructiveness had been used as a means to accomplish a benevolent purpose; or, in other words, that it had acted under the supremacy of moral sentiment and intellect, and we would approve of the transaction. If the world were created on the principle of Benevolence exclusively, no doubt the toothache could not exist; but, as pain does exist, Destructiveness has been given to place man in harmony with it, when used for a benevolent end.

To apply this illustration to the works of providence; I humbly suggest it as probable, that if we knew *thoroughly* the design and whole consequences of such institutions of the Creator, as are attended with pain, death, and disease, for example, we should find that Destructiveness was used as a *means*, under the guidance of Benevolence and Justice, to arrive at an end in harmony with the moral sentiments and intellect; in short, that no institution of the Creator has pure evil, or destructiveness alone, for its object. In judging of the divine institutions, the moral sentiments and intellect embrace the results of them to the *race*, while the propensities regard only the individual; and as the former are the higher powers, their dictates are of supreme authority in such questions. Further, when the operations of these institutions are sufficiently understood, they will be acknowledged to be beneficial for the individual also; although, when partially viewed, this may not at first appear to be the case.

The opposite of this doctrine, viz. that there are institutions of the Creator which have suffering for their exclusive object, is clearly untenable; for this would be ascribing malevolence to the Deity. As, however, the existence of pain is undeniable, it is equally impossible to believe that the world is arranged on the principle of Benevolence exclusively; and, with great submission, the view now presented reconciles the existence of Pain with that of Benevolence in a natural way, and the harmony of it with the constitution of the human mind, renders its soundness probable.

CHAPTER II.

OF THE CONSTITUTION OF MAN, AND ITS RELATIONS TO EXTERNAL OBJECTS.

Let us, then, consider the Constitution of Man, and the natural laws to which he is subjected, and endeavour to discover how far the external world is arranged with wisdom and benevolence, in regard to him. Bishop Butler, in the Preface to his Sermons, says, 'It is from considering the relations which the several appetites and passions in the inward frame have to each other, and, above all, the supremacy of reflection or conscience, that we get the idea of the system or constitution of human nature. And from the idea itself, it will as fully appear, that this our nature, *i. e.* constitution, is adapted to virtue, as from the idea of a watch it appears, that its nature, *i. e.* constitution or system, is adapted to measure time.

'Mankind has various instincts and principles of action, as brute creatures have; some leading most directly and immediately to the good of the community, and some most directly to private good.

'Man has several, which brutes have not; particularly reflection or conscience, an approbation of some principles or actions, and disapprobation of others.'

'Brutes obey their instincts or principles of action, according to certain rules; suppose, the constitution of their body, and the objects around them.'

'The generality of mankind also obey their instincts and principles, all of them, those propensities we call good, as well as the bad, according to the same rules, namely, the constitution of their body, and the external circumstances which they are in.'

'Brutes, in acting according to the rules before mentioned, their bodily constitution and circumstances, act suitably to *their whole nature.*

'Mankind also, in acting thus, would act suitably to their whole nature, if no more were to be said of man's nature than what has been now said; if that, as it is a true, were also a complete, adequate account of our nature.

'But that is not a complete account of man's nature. Somewhat further must be brought in to give us an adequate notion of it; namely, *that one of those principles of action, conscience, or reflection,* compared with the rest, as they all stand together in the nature of man, *plainly bears upon it marks of authority over all the rest, and claims the absolute direction of them all,* to allow or forbid their gratification;—a disapprobation on reflection being in itself a principle manifestly superior to a mere propension. And the conclusion is, that to allow no more to this superior principle or part of our nature, than to other parts; to let it govern and guide only occasionally, in common with the rest, as its turn happens to come, from the temper and circumstances one happens to be in; *this is not to act conformably to the constitution of man:* neither can any human creature be said to act conformably to his constitution of nature, unless he allows to that superior principle the absolute authority which is due to it.'—*Butler's Works*, vol. ii. *Preface.* The following Essay is founded on the principles here suggested.

SECTION I.

MAN CONSIDERED AS A PHYSICAL BEING.

The human body consists of bones, muscles, nerves, blood-vessels, besides organs of nutrition, of respiration, and of thought. These parts are all composed of physical elements, and, to a certain extent, are subjected to the physical laws of creation. By the law of gravitation, the body falls to the ground when unsupported, and is liable to be injured, like any frangible substance; by a chemical law, excessive cold freezes, and excessive heat dissipates its fluids; and life, in either case, is extinguished.

To discover the real effect of the physical laws of nature on human happiness, we would require to understand, 1st. The physical laws themselves, as revealed by mathematics, natural philosophy, natural history, and their subordinate branches; 2dly. The anatomical and physiological constitution of the human body; 3dly. The adaptation of the former to the latter. These expositions are necessary, to ascertain the extent to which it is possible for man to place himself in accordance with the physical laws, so as to reap advantage from them, and also to determine how far the sufferings which he endures, fail to be ascribed to their inevitable operation, and how far to his ignorance and infringement of them. To treat of these views in detail, would require separate volumes, and I therefore confine myself to a single instance as an illustration of the mode in which the investigation might be conducted.

By the law of gravitation, heavy bodies always tend towards the centre of the earth. Some of the advantages of this law are, that objects remain at rest when properly supported, so that men know where to find them when they are wanted for use; walls, when erected of sufficient thickness and perfectly perpendicular, stand firm and secure, so as to constitute edifices for the accommodation of man. Water descends from the clouds, from the roofs of houses, from streets and fields, and precipitates itself down the channels of rivers, turns mill-wheels in its course, and sets in motion the most stupendous and useful machinery; ships move steadily through the water with part of their hulls immersed, and part rising moderately above it, their masts and sails towering in the air to catch the inconstant breeze; and men are enabled to descend from heights, to penetrate by mines below the surface of the ground, and by diving-bells beneath that of the ocean.

To place man in harmony with this law, the Creator has bestowed on him bones, muscles, and nerves, constructed on the most perfect principles of mechanical science, which enable him to preserve his equilibrium, and to adapt his movements to its influence; also intellectual faculties, calculated to perceive the existence of the law, its modes of operation, the relation between it and himself, the beneficial consequences of observing this relation, and the painful results of infringing it.

Finally, when a person falls over a precipice, and is maimed or killed; when a ship springs a leak and sinks; or when a reservoir pond breaks down its banks and ravages a valley, we ought to trace the evil back to its cause, which will uniformly resolve itself into infringement of a natural law, and then endeavour to discover whether this infringement could or could not have been prevented, by a due exercise of the physical and mental powers bestowed by the Creator on man.

By pursuing this course, we shall arrive at sound conclusions concerning the adaptation of the human mind and body to the physical laws of creation. The subject, as I have said, is too extensive to be here prosecuted in detail, and I am incompetent, besides, to do it justice; but the more minutely any one inquires, the more firm will be his conviction, that in these relations admirable provision is made by the Creator for human happiness, and that the evils which arise from neglect of them, are attributable, to a great extent, to man's not adequately applying his powers to the promotion of his own enjoyment.

SECTION II.

MAN CONSIDERED AS AN ORGANISED BEING.

Man is an organised being, and subject to the organic laws. An organised being is one which derives its existence from a previously existing organised being, which subsists on food, which grows, attains maturity, decays, and dies. The first law, then, that must be obeyed, to render an organised being perfect in its kind, is that the germ, from which it springs, shall be complete in all its parts, and sound in its whole constitution. If we sow an acorn, in which some vital part has been destroyed altogether, the seedling plant, and the full grown oak, if it ever attain to maturity, will be deficient in the lineaments which were wanting in the embryo root; if we sow an acorn entire in its parts, but only half ripened or damaged, by damp or other causes, in its whole texture, the seedling oak will be feeble, and will probably die early. A similar law holds in regard to man. A second organic law is, that the organised being, the moment it is ushered into life, and so long as it continues to live, must be supplied with food, light, air, and other physical aliment requisite for its support, in due quantity, and of the kind best suited to its particular constitution. Obedience to this law is rewarded with a vigorous and healthy developement of its powers; and in animals, with a pleasing consciousness of existence and aptitude for the performance of their natural functions; disobedience to it is punished with feebleness, stinted growth, general imperfection, or death. A third organic law, applicable to man, is, that he shall duly exercise his organs, this condition being an indispensable requisite to health. The reward of obedience to this law, is enjoyment in the very act of exercising the functions, pleasing consciousness of existence, and the acquisition of numberless gratifications and advantages, of which labour, or the exercise of our powers, is the procuring means: disobedience is punished with derangement and sluggishness of the functions, with general uneasiness or positive pain, and with the denial of gratification to numerous faculties.

Directing our attention to the constitution of the human body, we perceive that the power of reproduction is bestowed on man, and also intellect, to enable him to discover and obey the conditions necessary for the transmission of a healthy organic frame to his descendants; that digestive organs are given to him for his nutrition, and innumerable vegetable and animal productions are placed around him, in wise relationship to these organs.

Without attempting to expound minutely the organic structure of man, or to trace in detail its adaptation to his external condition, I shall offer some observations in support of the proposition, that the due exercise of the osseous, muscular, and nervous systems, under the guidance of intellect and moral sentiment, and in accordance with the physical laws, contributes to human enjoyment; and, that neglect of this exercise, or an abuse of it, by carrying it to excess, or by conducting it in opposition to the moral, intellectual, or physical laws, is punished with pain.

The earth is endowed with the capability of producing an ample supply for all our wants, provided we expend muscular and nervous energy in its cultivation; while, in most climates, it refuses to produce if we withhold this labour and leave it waste. Further, the Creator has presented us with timber, metal, wool, and countless materials, which, by means of muscular power, may be converted into clothing, and all the luxuries of life. The fertility of the earth, and the demands of the body for food and clothing, are so benevolently adapted to each other, that, with rational restraint on population, a few hours' labour each day from every individual capable of labour, would suffice to furnish all with every commodity that could really add to enjoyment.

In the tropical regions of the globe, for example, where a high atmospheric temperature diminishes the quantum of muscular energy, the fertility and productiveness of the soil are increased in a like proportion, so that less labour suffices. Less labour, also, is required to provide habitations and raiment. In the colder latitudes, muscular energy is greatly increased, and there much higher demands are made upon it. The earth is more sterile, the rude winds require firmer fabrics to resist their violence, and the piercing frosts require a thicker covering to the body.

Further, the food afforded by the soil in each climate is admirably adapted to the maintenance of the organic constitution in health, and to the supply of the muscular energy requisite for the particular wants of the situation. In the Arctic Regions no farinaceous food ripens; but on putting the question to Dr. RICHARDSON, how he, accustomed to the bread and vegetables of the temperate regions, was able to endure the pure animal diet, which formed his only support on his expedition to the shores of the Polar Sea along with Captain FRANKLIN, he replied, that the effects of the extreme dry cold to which they were exposed, living, as they did, constantly in the open air, was to produce a desire for the most stimulating food they could obtain; that bread in such a climate was not only not desired, but comparatively impotent, as an article of diet; that pure animal food, and the fatter the better, was the only sustenance that maintained the tone of the corporeal system, but that when it was abundant (and the quantity required was much greater than in milder latitudes), a delightful vigour and buoyancy of body and mind were enjoyed, that rendered life highly agreeable. Now, in beautiful harmony with these wants of the human frame, these regions abound, during summer, in countless herds of deer, in rabbits, partridges, ducks, in short, in game of every description, and fish: and the flesh of these dried, constitutes delicious food in winter, when the earth is wrapped in one widespread covering of snow.

In Scotland, the climate is moist and cold, the greater part of the surface is mountainous, but admirably adapted for raising sheep and cattle, while a certain portion consists of fertile plains, fitted for farinaceous food. If the same law holds in this country, the diet of the people should consist of animal and farinaceous food, the former decidedly predominating. As we proceed to warmer latitudes, we find the soil and temperature of France less congenial to sheep and cattle, but more favourable to corn and wine; and the Frenchman inherits a native elasticity of body and mind, that enables him to flourish in vigour on less of animal food, than would be requisite to preserve the Scottish Highlander in a like gay and alert condition, in the recesses of his mountains. The plains of Hindostan are too hot for the sheep and ox, but produce rice and vegetable spices in prodigious abundance, and the native is healthy, vigorous and active, when supplied with rice and curry, and becomes sick, when obliged to live upon animal diet. He, also, is supplied with less muscular energy from this species of food, and his soil and climate require far less laborious exertion than those of Britain, Germany, or Russia.

So far, then, the external world appears to be wisely and benevolently adapted to the organic system of man, that is, to his nutrition, and to the developement and exercise of his corporeal organs; and the natural law appears to be, that all, if they desire to enjoy the pleasure attending sound and vigorous muscular and nervous systems, must expend in labour the energy which the Creator has infused into these organs. A wide choice is left open to man, as to the *mode* in which he shall exercise his nervous and muscular systems. The labourer, for example, digs the ground, and the squire engages in the chase. The penalty of neglecting this law is debility, bodily and mental, lassitude, imperfect digestion, disturbed sleep, bad health, and, if carried to a certain length, death. The penalty for over-exerting these systems is exhaustion, mental incapacity, the desire of strong artificial stimulants, such as ardent spirits, general insensibility, and grossness of feeling and perception, with disease and shortened life. Society has not recognised this law, and in consequence, the higher orders despise labour, and suffer the first penalty; while the lower orders are oppressed with toil, and undergo the second. The penalties serve to provide motives for obedience to the law, and whenever it is recognised, and the consequences are discovered to be inevitable, men will no longer shun labour as painful and ignominious, but resort to it as a source of pleasure, as well as to avoid the pains inflicted on those who neglect it.

SECTION III.

MAN CONSIDERED AS AN ANIMAL—MORAL—AND INTELLECTUAL BEING.

In the *third* place, man is an animal—moral—and intellectual being. To discover the adaptation of these parts of his nature to his external circumstances, we must first know what are his various animal, moral, and intellectual powers themselves. Phrenology gives us a view of them, drawn from observation; and as I have verified the inductions of that science, so as to satisfy myself that is the most complete and correct exposition of the Nature of Man which has yet been given, I adopt its classification of faculties as the basis of the subsequent observations. According to Phrenology, then, the Human Faculties are the following:

Order I. FEELINGS.

Genus I. PROPENSITIES—*Common to Man with the Lower Animals.*

1. AMATIVENESS;—Produces sexual love.
2. PHILOPROGENITIVENESS.—*Uses:* Love of offspring.—*Abuses:* Pampering and spoiling children.
3. CONCENTRATIVENESS.—*Uses:* It gives the desire for permanence in place, and for permanence of emotions and ideas in the mind.—*Abuses:* Aversion to move abroad; morbid dwelling on internal emotions and ideas, to the neglect of external impressions.
4. ADHESIVENESS.—*Uses:* Attachment; friendship, and society result from it.—*Abuses:* Clanship for improper objects, attachment to worthless individuals. It is generally large in women.
5. COMBATIVENESS.—*Uses:* Courage to meet danger, to overcome difficulties, and to resist attacks.—*Abuses:* Love of contention, and tendency to provoke and assault.
6. DESTRUCTIVENESS.—*Uses:* Desire to destroy noxious objects, and to kill for food. It is very discernible in carnivorous animals.—*Abuses:* Cruelty, desire to torment, tendency to passion, rage, harshness and severity in speech and writing.
7. CONSTRUCTIVENESS.—*Uses:* Desire to build and construct works of art.—*Abuses:* Construction of engines to injure or destroy, and fabrication of objects to deceive mankind.
8. ACQUISITIVENESS.—*Uses:* Desire to possess, and tendency to accumulate, articles of utility, to provide against want.—*Abuses:* Inordinate desire for property; selfishness; avarice.
9. SECRETIVENESS.—*Uses:* Tendency to restrain within the mind the various emotions and ideas that involuntarily present themselves, until the judgment has approved of giving them utterance; it also aids the artist and the actor in giving expression; and is an ingredient in prudence.—*Abuses:* Cunning, deceit, duplicity, lying, and, joined with Acquisitiveness, theft.

Genus II. SENTIMENTS.

I. *Sentiments common to Man with the Lower Animals.*

10. SELF-ESTEEM.—*Uses:* Self-interest, love of independence, personal dignity.—*Abuses:* Pride, disdain, overweening conceit, excessive selfishness, love of dominion.

11. **Love of Approbation.**—*Uses:* Desire of the esteem of others, love of praise, desire of fame or glory.—*Abuses:* Vanity, ambition, thirst for praise independent of praiseworthiness.
12. **Cautiousness.**—*Uses:* It gives origin to the sentiment of fear, the desire to shun danger, to circumspection; and it is an ingredient in prudence.—*Abuses:* Excessive timidity, poltroonery, unfounded apprehensions, despondency, melancholy.
13. **Benevolence.**—*Uses:* Desire of the happiness of others, universal charity, mildness of disposition, and a lively sympathy with the enjoyment of all animated beings.—*Abuses:* Profusion, injurious indulgence of the appetites and fancies of others, prodigality, facility of temper.

II. *Sentiments proper to Man.*

14. **Veneration.**—*Uses:* Tendency to worship, adore, venerate, or respect whatever is great and good; gives origin to the religious sentiment.—*Abuses:* Senseless respect for unworthy objects consecrated by time or situation, love of antiquated customs, abject subserviency to persons in authority, superstition.
15. **Hope.**—*Uses:* Tendency to expect and to look forward to the future with confidence and reliance; it cherishes faith.—*Abuses:* Credulity, absurd expectations of felicity not founded on reason.
16. **Ideality.**—*Uses:* Love of the beautiful and splendid, the desire of excellence, poetic feeling.—*Abuses:* Extravagance and absurd enthusiasm, preference of the showy and glaring to the solid and useful, a tendency to dwell in the regions of fancy, and to neglect the duties of life.
Wonder.—*Uses:* The desire of novelty, admiration of the new, the unexpected, the grand, and extraordinary.—*Abuses:* Love of the marvellous, astonishment,—*Note.* Veneration, Hope and Wonder, combined, give the tendency to religion; their abuses produce superstition and belief in false miracles, in prodigies, magic, ghosts, and all supernatural absurdities.
17. **Consciousness.**—*Uses:* It gives origin to the sentiment of justice, or respect for the rights of others, openness to conviction, the love of truth.—*Abuses:* Scrupulous adherence to noxious principles when ignorantly embraced, excessive refinement in the views of duty and obligation, excess in remorse, or self-condemnation.
18. **Firmness.**—*Uses:* Determination, perseverance, steadiness of purpose.—*Abuses:* Stubbornness, infatuation, tenacity in evil.

Order II. INTELLECTUAL FACULTIES.

Genus I. EXTERNAL SENSES.

FEELING or TOUCH.
TASTE.
SMELL.
HEARING.
LIGHT.

} *Uses:* To bring man into communication with external objects, and to enable him to enjoy them.—*Abuses:* Excessive indulgence in the pleasures arising from the senses, to the extent of impairing the organs and debilitating the mind.

Genus II. INTELLECTUAL FACULTIES—*which perceive existence.*

19. INDIVIDUALITY—Takes cognizance of existence and simple facts.
EVENTUALITY—Takes cognizance of occurrences and events.
20. FORM—Renders man observant of form.
21. SIZE—Renders man observant of dimensions, and aids perspective.
22. WEIGHT—Communicates the perception of momentum, weight, resistance, and aids equilibrium.
23. COLOURING—Gives perception of colours.

Genus III. INTELLECTUAL FACULTIES—*which perceive the relations of external objects.*

24. LOCALITY—Gives the idea of space and relative position.
25. ORDER—Communicates the love of physical arrangement.
26. TIME—Gives rise to the perception of duration.
27. NUMBER—Gives a turn for arithmetic and algebra.
28. TUNE—The sense of Melody arises from it.
29. LANGUAGE—Gives a facility in acquiring a knowledge of arbitrary signs to express thoughts—a facility in the use of them—and a power of inventing them.

Genus IV. REFLECTING FACULTIES—*which compare, judge, and discriminate.*

30. COMPARISON—Gives the power of discovering analogies and resemblances.
31. CAUSALITY—to trace the dependencies of phenomena, and the relation of cause and effect.
32. WIT—Gives the feeling and the ludicrous.
33. IMITATION—To copy the manners, gestures, and actions of others, and nature generally.

The first glance at these faculties suffices to show, that they are not all equal in excellence and elevation; that some are common to man with the lower animals; and others peculiar to man. In comparing the human mind, therefore, with its external condition, it becomes an object of primary importance to discover the relative subordination of these different orders of powers. If the Animal Faculties are naturally or necessarily supreme, then external nature, if it be wisely constituted, may be expected to bear direct reference, in its arrangements, to this supremacy. If the Moral and Intellectual Faculties hold the ascendency, then the constitution of external nature may be expected to be in harmony with them, when predominant. Let us attend to these questions.

SECTION IV.

THE FACULTIES OF MAN COMPARED WITH EACH OTHER; OR THE SUPREMACY OF THE MORAL SENTIMENTS AND INTELLECT.

According to the phrenological theory of human nature, the faculties are divided into Propensities common to man with the lower animals, Sentiments common to man, with the lower animals, Sentiments proper to man, and intellect. Every faculty stands in a definite relation to certain external objects;—when it is internally active it desires these objects;—when they are presented to it they excite it to activity, and delight it with agreeable sensations. Human happiness and misery are resolved into the gratification or denial of gratification of one or more of our active faculties, before described, of the external senses, and the feelings connected with our bodily frame. The faculties, in themselves, are mere instincts; the moral sentiments and intellect are higher instincts than the animal propensities. Every faculty is good in itself, but all are liable to abuse.

Their manifestations are right only when directed by *enlightened* intellect and moral sentiment. In maintaining the *supremacy* of the moral sentiments and intellect, I *do not* consider them sufficient to direct conduct by *their mere instinctive suggestions*. To fit them to discharge this important duty, *they must be illuminated by knowledge of science and of moral and religious duty ;* but whenever their dictates, thus enlightened, oppose the solicitations of the propensities, *the latter must yield*, otherwise, *by the constitution of external nature*, evil will inevitably ensue. This is what I mean by nature being constituted in harmony with the supremacy of the moral sentiments and intellect. Let us consider the faculties themselves.

The first three propensities, Amativeness, Philoprogenitiveness, and Adhesiveness, or the group of the domestic affections, desire a conjugal partner, offspring, and friends; the obtaining of these affords them delight,—the removal of them occasions pain. But to render an individual happy, the whole faculties must be gratified harmoniously, or at least the gratification of one or more must not offend any of the others. For example, suppose the group of the domestic affections to be highly interested in an individual, and strongly to desire to form an alliance with him, but that the person so loved is improvident and immoral, and altogether an object which the faculties of Self-esteem, Love of Approbation, Benevolence, Veneration, Conscientiousness, and Intellect, if left dispassionately to survey his qualities, could not approve of; then, if an alliance be formed with him, under the ungovernable impulses of the former faculties, bitter days of repentance must necessarily follow, when these begin to languish, and the latter faculties receive offence from his qualities. If, on the other hand, the domestic affections are guided by intellect to an object pleasing to the latter powers, these themselves will be gratified, they will double the delights afforded by the former faculties, and render the enjoyment permanent.

The great distinction between the animal faculties and the powers proper to man, is, that the object of the former is the preservation of the individual himself, or his family; while the latter have the welfare of others, and our duties to God, as their ends. Even the domestic affections, amiable and respectable as they undoubtedly are when combined with the moral feelings, have self as their object. The love of children, springing from Philoprogenitiveness, when acting alone, is the same in kind as that of the miser for his gold; an intense interest in the object, for the sake of the gratification it affords to his own mind, without regard for the object on its own account. This truth is recognised by Sir WALTER SCOTT. He says 'Elspat's ardent, *though selfish affection* for her son, *incapable of being qualified by a regard for the true interests of the unfortunate object of her attachment, resembled the instinctive fondness of the animal race for their offspring;* and, *diving little farther into futurity than one of the inferior creatures, she only felt that to be separated from Hamish was to die.*'*

In man, this faculty generally acts along with Benevolence, and a disinterested desire of the happiness of the child mingles along with, and elevates the mere instinct of, Philoprogenitiveness; but the sources of these two affections are different, their degrees vary in different persons, and their ends also are dissimilar.

The same observation applies to the affection proceeding from Adhesiveness. When this faculty acts alone, it desires, for its own satisfaction, a friend to love; but, if Benevolence do not act along with it, it cares nothing for the happiness of that friend, except in so far as his welfare may be necessary to its own gratification. The horse feels melancholy when his companion is removed; but the feeling appears to be one of uneasiness at the absence of an ob-

---

* Chronicles of Cannongate, vol. i. p. 281.

ject which gratified his Adhesiveness. His companion may have been led to a richer pasture, and introduced to more agreeable society; yet this does not assuage the distress suffered by him at his removal; his tranquillity, in short, is restored only by time causing the activity of Adhesiveness to subside, or by the substitution of another object on which it may exert itself. In human nature, the effect of the faculty, when acting singly, is the same; and this accounts for the fact of the almost total indifference of many persons who were really attached, by Adhesiveness, to each other, when one falls into misfortune, and becomes a disagreeable object to the Self-esteem and Love of Approbation of the other. Suppose two persons, elevated in rank, and possessed of affluence, to have each Adhesiveness, Self-esteem, and Love of Approbation large, with Benevolence and Conscientiousness moderate, it is obvious that, while both are in prosperity, they may really like each other's society, and feel a reciprocal attachment, because there will be mutual sympathy in their Adhesiveness, and the Self-eeteem and Love of Approbation of each will be gratified by the rank and circumstances of his friend; but imagine one of them to fall into misfortune, and to cease to be an object gratifying to Self-esteem and Love of Approbation; suppose that he becomes a poor friend instead of a rich and influential one, the harmony between their selfish faculties will be broken, and then Adhesiveness in the one who remains rich will transfer its affection to another individual who may gratify it, and also supply agreeable sensations to Self-esteem and Love of Approbation,—to a genteel friend, in short, who will look well in the eye of the world.

Much of this conduct occurs in society, and the whining complaint is very ancient, that the storms of adversity disperse friends just as the winter winds strip leaves from the forest that gaily adorned it in the sunshine of summer; and many moral sentences are pointed, and episodes finely turned, on the selfishness and corruption of poor human nature. But such friendships were attachments founded on the lower feelings, which, by their constitution, are selfish, and the desertion complained of is the fair and legitimate result of the principles on which both parties acted during the gay hours of prosperity. If we look at the head of SHERIDAN, we shall perceive large Adhesiveness, Self-esteem, and, Love of Approbation, with deficient reflecting organs, and moderate Conscientiousness. He has large Individuality, Comparison, Secretiveness, and Imitation, which gave him talents for observation and display. When these earned him a brilliant reputation, he was surrounded by friends, and he himself probably felt attachment in return. But his deficient morality prevented him from loving his friends with a true, disinterested, and honest regard; he abused their kindness, and, as he sunk into poverty and wretchedness, and ceased to be an honour to them, or to excite their Love of Approbation, they almost all deserted him. But the whole connexion was founded on selfish principles; SHERIDAN honoured them, and they flattered SHERIDAN; and the abandonment was the natural consequence of the cessation of gratification to their selfish feelings. I shall by-and-by point out the sources of a loftier and a purer friendship, and its effects.

To proceed with the propensities: Combativeness and Destructiveness also are in their nature purely selfish. If aggression is committed against us, Combativeness draws the sword and repels the attack: Destructiveness inflicts vengeance for the offence; both feelings are obviously the very opposite of benevolent. I do not say, that, in themselves, they are despicable or sinful; on the contrary, they are necessary, and when legitimately employed, highly useful; but still self is the object of their supreme regard.

The next organ is Acquisitiveness; and self is eminently its object. It desires blindly to possess, is pleased with accumulating, and suffers great uneasiness in being deprived of its objects. It is highly useful, like all the other faculties, for even Benevolence cannot give away until Acquisitiveness have acquired. There are friendships, particularly among mercantile men, founded on Adhesiveness and Acquisitiveness, just as in fashionable life they are founded on Adhesiveness and Love of Approbation. Two individuals fall into a course of dealing, by which each reaps profit by transactions with the other: this leads to intimacy, and Adhesiveness probably mingles its influence, and produces a feeling of actual attachment. The moment, however, that the Acquisitiveness of the one suffers the least inroad from that of the other, and their interests clash, they are apt, if no higher principle unite them, to become bitter enemies. It is probable that, while these fashionable and commercial friendships last, the parties may profess great reciprocal esteem and regard, and that, when a rupture takes place, the one who is depressed, or disobliged, may recall these expressions and charge them as hypocritical; but they really were not so: each probably felt from Adhesiveness and gratified Love of Approbation something which he coloured over, and perhaps believed to be disinterested friendship; but if each would honestly probe his own conscience, he would be obliged to acknowledge that the whole basis of the connexion was selfish; and hence, that the result is just what every man ought to expect, who places his reliance for happiness chiefly on the lower propensities.

Secretiveness is also selfish in its nature; for it suppresses feelings that might injure us with other individuals, and desires to find out secrets that may enable its possessor to guard self against hostile plots or designs. In itself it does not desire, in any respect, the benefit of others.

Self-esteem is, in its very essence and name, selfish; it is the love of ourselves, and the esteem of ourselves *par excellence.*

Love of Approbation, although many think otherwise, is

also in itself a purely selfish feeling. Its real desire is applause to ourselves, to be esteemed ourselves, and if it prompt us to do services, or to say agreeable things to others, it is not from love of them, but purely for the sake of obtaining self-gratification.

Suppose, for example, we are acquainted with a person who has committed an error in some public duty, who has done or said something that the public disapprove of, and which we see to be really wrong, Benevolence and Conscientiousness would prompt us to lay before our freind the very head and front of his offending, and conjure him to forsake his error, and publicly make amends :—Love of Approbation, on the other hand, would either render us averse to speak to him on the subject, lest he should be offended, or prompt us to extenuate his fault, and represent it as either positively no error at all, or as extremely trivial. If we analyze the motive which prompts to this course, we shall find that it is not love of our friend, or consideration for his welfare, but fear lest, by our presenting to him disagreeable truths, he should feel offended at us, and deprive us of the gratification afforded to our Love of Approbation by his good opinion : in short, the motive is purely selfish.

Another illustration occurs. A manufacturer in a country town, having acquired a considerable fortune by trade, applied part of it in building a princely mansion, which he furnished in the richest and most expensive style of fashion. He asked his customers, near and distant, to visit him when calling on business, and led them into a dining-room or drawing-room that absolutely dazzled them with its magnificence. This excited their wonder and curiosity, which was precisely the effect he desired ; he then led them over his whole apartments, and displayed before them his grandeur and taste. In doing so, he imagined that he was conferring a high pleasure on them, and filling tneir minds with an intense admiration of his greatness; but the real effect was very different. The motive of his conduct was not love of them, or regard for their happiness or welfare; it was not Benevolence to others that prompted him to build the palace; it was not Veneration, nor was it Conscientiousness. The fabric sprung from Self-esteem and Love of Approbation combined, no doubt, with considerable Intellect and Ideality. In leading his humble brethren in trade through the princely halls, over the costly carpets, and amidst the gilding, burnishing, and rich array, that everywhere met their eyes, he exulted in the consciousness of his own importance, and asked for their admiration, not as an expression of respect for any real benefits conferred upon them, but as the much relished food of his own selfish vanity.

Let us attend, in the next place, to the effect of this display on those to whom it was addressed. To gain their esteem or affection, it was necessary to manifest towards them real Benevolence, real regard, and impartial justice; in short, to cause another individual to love us, we must make him the object of the moral sentiments, which have his good and happiness for their end. Here, however, these were not the inspiring motives of the conduct, and the want of them would be instinctively felt. The customers, who possessed the least shrewdness, would ascribe the whole exhibition to the vanity of the owner, and they would either pity or hate him; if their own moral sentiments predominated, they would pity; if their Self-esteem and Love of Approbation were paramount, these would be offended at his assumed superiority, and would rouse Destructiveness to hate him. It would only be the silliest and the vainest who would be at all gratified; and their satisfaction would arise from the feeling, that they could now return to their own circle, and boast how great a friend they had, and in how grand a style they had been entertained, —this display being a direct gratification of their own Self-esteem and Love of Approbation, by their identifying themselves with him. Even this pleasure could be reaped only where the admirer was so humble in rank as to entertain no idea of rivalship, and so limited in intellect and sentiments as not to perceive the worthlessness of the qualities by which he was captivated.

In like manner, when persons, even of more sense than the manufacturer here alluded to, give entertainments to their friends, they sometimes fail in their object from the same cause. They wish to show off themselves as their leading motive, much more than to confer real happiness upon their acquaintances; and, by the irreversible law of human nature, this must fail in exciting good will and pleasure in the minds of those to whom it is addressed, because it disagreeably affects their Self-esteem and Love of Approbation. In short, to be really successful in gratifying our friends, we must keep our own selfish faculties in due subordination, and pour out copious streams of real kindness from the higher sentiments, animated and elevated by intellect; and all who have experienced the heartfelt joy and satisfaction attending an entertainment conducted on this principle, will never quarrel with the homeliness of the fare, or feel uneasy about the absence of fashion in the service.

Cautiousness is the next faculty, and is a sentiment instituted to protect self from danger, and has clearly a regard to individual safety as its primary object.

This terminates the list of the feelings common to man with the lower animal,* and which, as we have seen, have self preservation as their leading objects. They are given for the protection and advantage of our animal nature, and, when duly regulated, are highly useful, and also respectable, viewed with reference to that end; but they are sources

---

* Benevolence is stated in the works on Phrenology as common to man with the lower animals; but in them it appears to produce rather passive meekness and good nature, than actual desire for each other's happiness. In the human race, this last is its proper function; and, viewed in this light, I here treat of it as exclusively a human faculty.

of innumerable evils when allowed to usurp the ascendency over the moral faculties, and to become the leading springs of our social intercourse.

I proceed to notice the moral sentiments which constitute the proper human faculties, and to point out their objects and relations.

Benevolence has no reference to self. It desires purely and disinterestedly the happiness of its object; it loves for the sake of the person beloved; if he be well, and the sunbeams of prosperity shine warmly around him, it exults and delights in his felicity. It desires a diffusion of joy, and renders the feet swift and the arm strong in the cause of charity and love.

Veneration also has no reference to self. It looks up with a pure and elevated emotion to the being to whom it is directed, whether God or our fellow-men, and delights in the contemplation of their venerable and admirable qualities. It desires to find out excellence, and to dwell and feed upon it, and renders self lowly, humble, and submissive.

Hope spreads its gay wing in the boundless regions of futurity. It desires good, and expects it to come; " it incites us to aim at a good which we can live without;" its influence is soft, soothing, and happy; but self is not its direct or particular object.

Ideality delights in perfection from the pure pleasure of contemplating it. So far as it is concerned, the picture, the statue, the landscape, or the mansion, on which it abides with intensest rapture, will be as pleasing, although the property of another, as if all its own. It is a spring that is touched by the beautiful wherever it exists; and hence its means of enjoyment are as unbounded as the universe is extensive.

Wonder seeks the new and the striking, and is delighted with change; but there is no desire of appropriation to self in its longings.

Conscientiousness stands in the midway between self and other individuals. It is a regulator of our animal feelings, and points out the limit which they must not pass. It desires to do to another as we would have another to do to us, and thus is a guardian of the welfare of our fellow men, while it sanctions and supports our personal feelings within the bounds of a due moderation. It is a noble feeling; and the mere consciousness of its being bestowed upon us, ought to bring home to our minds an intense conviction that the Author of the universe is at once wise and just.

Intellect is universal in its application. It may become the handmaid of any of the faculties; it may devise a plan to murder or to bless, to steal or to bestow, to rear up or to destroy; but, as its proper use is to observe the different objects of creation, to mark their relations, and direct the propensities and sentiments to their proper and legitimate enjoyments, it has a boundless sphere of activity, and, when properly exercised and applied, is a source of high and inexhaustible delight.

Keeping in view the great difference now pointed out between the animal and properly human faculties, the reader will perceive that three consequences follow from the constitution of these powers: *First*, All the faculties, when in excess, are insatiable, and, from the constitution of the world, never can be satisfied. They indeed may be soon satisfied on any particular occasion. Food will soon fill the stomach; indulgence will speedily assuage Amativeness; success in a speculation will render Acquisitiveness quiescent for the moment: a triumph will satisfy for the time Self-esteem and Love of Approbation; a long concert will fatigue Tune; and, too long a discourse afflict Causality. But after repose they will all *renew their solicitations*. They must all therefore be regulated; and, in particular, the lower propensities, from having self as their primary object, and being blind to consequences, do not set limits to their own indulgence; and hence lead to misery to the individual, and injury to society, when allowed to exceed the limits prescribed by the superior sentiments and intellect.

As this circumstance attending the propensities is of great practical importance, I shall make a few observations in elucidation of it. The births and lives of children depend upon circumstances, over which unenlightened men have but a limited control : and hence an individual, whose supreme happiness springs from the gratification of Philoprogenitiveness will, by the mere predominance of that propensity, be led to neglect or infringe the natural laws, on which the lives and welfare of children depend, and which can be observed only by active moral and intellectual faculties. Hence he will be in constant danger of anguish and disappointment, by the removal of his children, or by their undutiful conduct and immoral behaviour. Besides, Philoprogenitiveness, acting along with Self-esteem and Love of Approbation, would, in each parent, desire that *his* children should possess the highest rank, the greatest wealth, and be distinguished for the most splendid talents. Now the highest, the greatest, and the most splendid of any qualities, necessarily imply the existence of inferior degrees, and are not attainable except by one. The animal faculties, therefore, must be restrained in their desires, and directed to their objects by the human faculties, by the sentiments of Conscientiousness, Benevolence, Veneration, and Intellect, otherwise they will inevitably lead to disappointment. In like manner, Acquisitiveness desires wealth, and, as nature affords only a certain number of quarters of grain annually, a certain portion of cattle, of fruit, of flax, and other articles, from which food, clothing, and wealth, are manufactured ; and as this quantity, divided equally among all the members of a state, would afford but a moderate portion to each, it is self-evident that, if all desire to acquire and possess a large amount, ninety-nine out of the hundred must be disappointed. This disappointment, from the very constitution of nature, is inevitable to the greater number; and when individuals form schemes of aggrandisement, originating from desires communicated by the animal faculties alone, they would do well to keep this law of nature in view. When we look around, we see how few make rich; how few succeed in accomplishing all their lofty anticipations for the advancement of their children; how few attain the summit of ambition, compared with the multitudes who fall short. Love of Approbation and Self-esteem, when unregulated, desire the highest station of ambition; but, as these faculties exist in all men, and only one can be greatest, they will prompt one man to defeat the gratification of another. All this arises, not from error and imperfection in the institutions of the Creator, but from blindness in men to their own nature, to the nature of external objects, and to the relations established between these; in short, blindness to the principles of the divine administration of the world.

Secondly. The animal propensities being inferior in their nature to the human faculties, their gratifications, when not approved of by the latter, leave a painful feeling of discontent and dissatisfaction in the mind, occasioned by the secret disclaimation of their excessive action by the higher feelings. Suppose, for example, a young person to set out in life, with the idea that the great object of existence is to acquire wealth, to rear and provide for a family, and to attain honour and distinction among men; all these desires spring from the propensities alone. Imagine him to rise early and sit up late, to put forth all the energies of a powerful mind in buying, selling, and making rich, and that he is successful: it is obvious, that, in prompting to this course of action, Benevolence, Veneration, and Conscientiousness, had no share; and that, in pursuing it, they have not received direct and intended gratification; they would have anxiously and wearily watched the animal faculties, longing for the hour when they were to say

Enough; their whole occupation, in the mean time, being to restrain them from such gross extravagances as would have defeated their own ends. In the domestic circle, again, a spouse and children would gratify Philoprogenitiveness and Adhesiveness, and their advancement would please Self-esteem and Love of Approbation; but here also the moral sentiments would act the part of mere spectators and sentinels to impose restraints; they would receive no direct enjoyment, and would not be recognised as the fountain of the conduct. In the pursuit of honour, suppose an office of dignity and power, or high rank in society, the mainsprings of exertion would still be Self-esteem and Love of Approbation, and the moral sentiments would be compelled to wait in tiresome vacuity, without having their energies called directly into play, so as to give them full scope in their legitimate sphere.

Suppose, then, this individual to have reached the evening of life, and to look back on the pleasures and pains of his past existence, he must feel that there has been vanity and vexation of spirit,—the want of a satisfying portion; and for this sufficient reason, that the highest of his faculties have been all along scarcely employed. In estimating, also, the real affection and esteem of mankind which he has gained, he will find it to be small or great in exact proportion to the degree in which he has manifested, in his habitual conduct, the lower or the higher faculties. If society has seen him selfish in his pursuit of wealth, selfish in his domestic affections, selfish in his ambition; although he may have gratified all these feelings without positive encroachment on the rights of others, they will still look coldly on him, they will feel no glow of affection towards him, no elevated respect, no sincere admiration; he will see and feel this, and complain bitterly that all is vanity and vexation of spirit. But the fault has been his own; love, esteem, and sincere respect, arise, by the Creator's laws, not from contemplating the manifestations of plodding, selfish faculties, but only from the display of Benevolence, Veneration, and Justice, as the motives and end of our conduct; and the individual supposed has reaped the natural and legitimate produce of the soil which he cultivated, and eaten the fruit which he has reared.

Thirdly. The higher feelings, when directed by enlightened intellect, have a boundless scope for gratification; their least indulgence is delightful, and their highest activity is bliss; they cause no repentance, leave no void, but render life a scene at once of peaceful tranquillity and sustained felicity; and, what is of much importance, conduct proceeding from their dictates carries in its train the highest gratification to the animal propensities themselves, of which the latter are susceptible. At the same time, it must be observed, that the sentiments err, and lead also to evil, when not regulated by enlightened intellect; that intellect in its turn must give due weight to the existence and desires of both the propensities and sentiments, as elements in the human constitution, before it can arrive at sound conclusions regarding conduct; and that rational actions and true happiness flow from the gratification of all the faculties *in harmony* with each other; the sentiments and intellect bearing the directing sway.

This proposition may be shortly illustrated. Imagine an individual to commence life, with the thorough conviction that the higher sentiments are the superior powers, and that they ought to be the sources of his actions, the first effect would be to cause him to look habitually outward on other men and on his Creator, instead of looking inward on himself as the object of his highest and chief regard. Benevolence would shed on his mind the conviction, that there are other human beings as dear to the Creator as he, as much entitled to enjoyment as he, and that his duty is to seek no gratification to himself which is to injure them; but, on the contrary, to act so as to confer on them, by his daily exertions, all the services in his power. Veneration

would give a strong feeling of reliance on the power and
wisdom of God, that such conduct would conduce to the
highest gratification of all his faculties; it would add also
an habitual respect for his fellow men, as beings deserving
his regard, and to whose reasonable wishes he was bound
to yield a willing and sincere obedience. Lastly, Conscientiousness would prompt him to apply the scales of rigid
justice to his animal desires, and to curb and restrain each
so as to prevent the slightest infraction on what is due to
his fellow men.

Let us trace, then, the operation of these principles in
ordinary life. Suppose a friendship formed by such an individual: his first and fundamental principle is Benevolence, which inspires with a sincere, pure, and disinterested regard for his friend; he desires his welfare for his
friend's sake; next Veneration reinforces this love by the
secret and grateful acknowledgment which it makes to
Heaven for the joys conferred upon the mind by this pure
emotion, and also by the habitual deference which it inspires towards our friend himself, rendering us ready to
yield where compliance is becoming, and curbing our selfish feelings when these would intrude by interested or
arrogant pretensions on his enjoyment; and thirdly, Conscientiousness, ever on the watch, proclaims the duty of
making no unjust demands on the Benevolence of our
friend, but of limiting our whole intercourse with him on
an interchange of kindness, good offices, and reciprocal
affection. Intellect, acting along with these principles,
would point out, as an indispensable requisite to such an
attachment, that the friend himself should be so far under
the influence of the sentiments, as to be able, in some degree, to meet them; for, if he were immoral, selfish, vainly
ambitious, or, in short, under the habitual influence of the
propensities, the sentiments could not love and respect him;
they might pity him as unfortunate, but love him they could

not, because this is impossible by the very laws of their constitution.

Let us now attend to the degree in which such a friendship would gratify the lower propensities. In the first place, how would Adhesiveness exult and rejoice in such an attachment! It would be overpowered with delight, because, if the intellect were convinced that the friend habitually acknowledged the supremacy of the higher sentiments, Adhesiveness might pour forth all its ardour, and cling to its object with the closest bonds of affection. The friend would not encroach on us for evil, because his Benevolence and Justice would oppose this; he would not lay aside restraint, and break through the bonds of affection by undue familiarity, because Veneration would forbid this; he would not injure us in our name, person, or reputation, because Conscientiousness, Veneration, and Benevolence, all combined, would prevent such conduct. Here then Adhesiveness, freed from the fear of evil, from the fear of deceit, from the fear of dishonour, because a friend who should habitually act thus, could not possibly fall into dishonour, would be at liberty to take its deepest draught of affectionate attachment; it would receive a gratification which it is impossible it could attain, while acting in combination with the purely selfish faculties. What delight, too, would such a friendship afford to Self-esteem and Love of Approbation! There would be an internal approval of ourselves, that would legitimately gratify Self-esteem, because it would arise from a survey of pure motives, and just and benevolent actions. Love of Approbation also, would be gratified in the highest degree; for every act of affection, every expression of esteem, from such a friend, would be so purified by Benevolence, Veneration, and Conscientiousness, that it would form the legitimate food on which Love of Approbation might feast and be satisfied; it would fear no hollowness beneath, no tattling

MORAL SENTIMENTS AND INTELLECT. 45

in absence, no secret smoothing over for the sake of mere effect, no envyings, and no jealousies. In short, friendship founded on the higher sentiments, as the ruling motives, would delight the mind with gladness and sunshine, and gratify all the faculties, animal, moral, and intellectual, in *harmony* with each other.

By this illustration, the reader will understand more clearly what I mean by the harmony of the faculties. The fashionable and commercial friendships of which I spoke, gratified the propensities of Adhesiveness, Love of Approbation, Self-esteem, and Acquisitiveness, but left out, as fundamental principles, all the higher sentiments;—there was, therefore, a want of harmony in these instances, an absence of full satisfaction, an uncertainty and changeableness, which gave rise to only a mixed and imperfect enjoyment while the friendship lasted, and to a feeling of painful disappointment, and of vanity and vexation, when a rupture occurred. The error, in such cases, consists in founding attachment on the lower faculties, seeing they, by themselves, are not calculated to form a stable basis of affection, instead of building it on them and the higher sentiments, which afford a foundation for real, lasting, and satisfactory friendship. In complaining of the vanity and vexation of attachments springing from the lower faculties exclusively, we are like men who should try to build a pyramid on its smaller end, and then, lament the hardness of their fate, and speak of the unkindness of Providence, when it fell. A similar analysis of all other pleasures founded on the animal propensities chiefly, would give similar results. In short, happiness must be viewed by men as connected inseparably with the exercise of the three great classes of faculties, the moral sentiments and intellect exercising the directing and controlling sway, before it can be permanently attained.

SECTION V.

THE FACULTIES OF MAN COMPARED WITH EXTERNAL OBJECTS.

Having considered man as a *physical* being, and briefly adverted to the adaptation of his constitution to the physical laws of creation; having viewed him as an *organised* being, and traced the relations of his organic structure to his external circumstances; having taken a rapid survey of his *faculties*, as an animal, moral, and intellectual being,—with their uses and the forms of their abuse,—and having contrasted these faculties with each other, and discovered the supremacy of the moral sentiments and intellect, I proceed to compare his faculties with *external objects*, in order to discover what provision has been made for their gratification.

1. Amativeness is a feeling obviously necessary to the continuance of the species; and one which, properly regulated, is not offensive to reason;—opposite sexes exist to provide for its gratification.*
2. Philoprogenitiveness is given,—and offspring exist.
3. Concentrativeness is conferred,—and the other faculties are its objects.
4. Adhesiveness is given,—and country and friends exist.
5. Combativeness is bestowed,—and physical and moral obstacles exist, requiring courage to meet and subdue them.
6. Destructiveness is given,—and man is constituted with a carnivorous stomach, and animals to be killed and eaten exist. Besides, the whole combinations of creation are in a state of decay and renovation. In the animal kingdom almost every species of creatures is the prey of some other; and the faculty of Destructiveness places the human mind in harmony with this order of creation. Destruction makes way for renovation,

---

* The nature and sphere of activity of the phrenological faculties is explained at length in the 'System of Phrenology,' to which I beg to refer. Here I can only indicate general ideas.

and the act of renovation furnishes occasion for the activity of our powers; and activity is pleasure. That destruction is a natural institution is unquestionable. Not only has nature taught the spider to construct a web for the purpose of ensnaring flies, that it may devour them, and constituted beasts of prey with carnivorous teeth, but she has formed even plants, such as the Drosera, to catch and kill flies, and use them for food. Destructiveness serves also to give weight to indignation, a most important defensive as well as vindicatory purpose. It is a check upon undue encroachment, and tends to constrain mankind to pay regard to the rights and feelings of each other. When properly regulated, it is an able assistant to justice.

7. CONSTRUCTIVENESS is given,—and materials for constructing artificial habitations, raiment, ships, and various other fabrics that add to the enjoyment of life, have been provided to give it scope.

8. ACQUISITIVENESS is bestowed,—and property exists capable of being collected, preserved, and applied to use.

9. SECRETIVENESS is given,—and our faculties possess internal activity requiring to be restrained, until fit occasions and legitimate objects present themselves for their gratification; which restraint is rendered not only possible but agreeable, by the propensity in question. While we suppress and confine one feeling within the limits of our own consciousness, we exercise and gratify another in the very act of doing so.

10. SELF-ESTEEM is given,—and we have an individual existence and individual interests, as its objects.

11. LOVE OF APPROBATION is bestowed,—and we are surrounded by our fellow men, whose good opinion is the object of its desire.

12. CAUTIOUSNESS is given,—and it is admirably adapted to the nature of the external world. The human body is combustible, is liable to be destroyed by violence, to suffer injury from extreme wet and winds, &c.; and it is necessary for us to be habitually watchful to avoid these sources of calamity. Accordingly, Cautiousness is bestowed on us as an ever watchful sentinel, constantly whispering, 'Take care.' There is ample scope for the legitimate and pleasurable exercise of all our faculties, without running into these evils, provided we know enough, and are watchful enough; and, therefore, Cautiousness is not overwhelmed with inevitable terrors. It serves merely as a warder to excite us to beware of sudden and unexpected

danger; it keeps the other faculties at their post, by furnishing a stimulus to them to observe and trace consequences, that safety may be insured; and, when these other faculties do their duty in proper form, the impulses of Cautiousness are not painful, but the reverse: they communicate a feeling of internal security and satisfaction, expressed by the motto *Semper paratus;* and hence this faculty appears equally benevolent in its design, as the others which we have contemplated.

Here, then, we perceive a beautiful provision made for supporting the activity of, and affording legitimate gratification to, the lower propensities. These powers are conferred on us clearly to support our animal nature, and to place us in harmony with the external objects of creation. So far from their being injurious or base in themselves, they possess the dignity of utility, and the estimable quality of being sources of high enjoyment, when legitimately indulged. The phrenologist, therefore, would never seek to extirpate, nor to weaken them too much. He desires only to see their excesses controlled, and their exercise directed in accordance with the great institutions and designs of the Creator.

The next class of faculties is that of the moral sentiments proper to man. These are the following:

BENEVOLENCE is given,—and sentient and intelligent beings are created, whose happiness we are able to increase, thereby affording it its scope and delight. It is an error to imagine, that creatures in misery are the only objects of benevolence, and that it has no function but the excitement of pity. It is a wide-spreading fountain of generous feeling, desiring for its gratification not only the removal of pain, but the maintenance and augmentation of positive enjoyment; and the happier it can render its objects, the more complete are its satisfaction and delight. Its exercise, like that of all the other faculties, is a source of great pleasure to the individual himself; and nothing can be conceived more admirably adapted for affording it scope, than the system of creation exhibited on earth. From the nature of the human faculties, each individual, without injuring himself, has it in his power to confer prodigious benefits, or, in other words, to pour forth the most copious streams of benevolence on others, by legitimately gratifying their Adhesiveness, Constructiveness, Acquisitiveness, Love of Approbation, Self-esteem, Cautiousness, Veneration, Hope, Ideality, Conscientiousness, and their Knowing and Reflecting Faculties.

VENERATION.—The legitimate object of this faculty is the Divine Being; and I assume here, that phrenology enables us to demonstrate the existence of God. The very essay in which I am now engaged, is an attempt at an exposition of some of his attributes, as manifested in this world. If we shall find contrivance, wisdom, and benevolence in his works, unchangeableness, and no shadow of turning in his laws; perfect harmony in each department of creation, and shall discover that the evils which afflict us are much less the direct objects of his arrangements than the consequences of ignorant neglect of institutions calculated for our enjoyment,—then we shall acknowledge in the Divine Being an object whom we may love with our whole soul, reverence with the deepest emotions of veneration, and on whom Hope and Conscientiousness may repose with a perfect and unhesitating reliance. The exercise of this sentiment is in itself a great positive enjoyment, when the object is in harmony with all our other faculties. Further, its activity disposes us to yield obedience to the Creator's laws, the object of which is our own happiness; and hence its exercise is in the highest degree provided for. Revelation unfolds the character and intentions of God where reason cannot penetrate, but its doctrines do not fall within the limits prescribed to this Essay.

HOPE is given,—and our understanding, by discovering the laws of nature, is enabled to penetrate into the future. This sentiment then, is gratified by the absolute reliance which Causality warrants us to place on the stability and wisdom of the divine arrangements; its legitimate exercise, in reference to this life is to give us a vivifying faith, that while we suffer evil, we are undergoing a chastisement for having neglected the institutions of the Creator, the object of which punishment is to force us back into the right path. Revelation presents to Hope the certainty of a life to come; and directs all our faculties in points of Faith.

IDEALITY is bestowed,—and not only is external nature invested with the most exquisite loveliness, but a capacity for moral and intellectual refinement is given to us, by which we may rise in the scale of excellence, and at every step of our progress reap direct enjoyment from this sentiment. Its constant desire is for ' something more excellent still :' in its own immediate impulses it is delightful, and external nature and our own faculties respond to its call.

WONDER prompts to admiration, and desires something new. When we contemplate man endowed with intellect to discover a Diety and to comprehend his works, we cannot, doubt of Wonder being provided with objects for its intensest exercise; and when we view him placed in a world where all old things are constantly passing away, and a system of renovation is incessantly proceeding, we see at once how vast a provision is made for the gratification of his desire of novelty, and how admirably it is calculated to impel his other faculties to activity.

CONSCIENTIOUSNESS exists,—and it is necessary to prove that all the divine institutions are founded in justice, to afford it full satisfaction. This is a point which many regard as involved in much obscurity: I shall endeavour in this Essay to lift the veil, for to me justice appears to flow through every divine institution.

One difficulty, in regard to Conscientiousness, long appeared inexplicable; it was, how to reconcile with Benevolence the institution by which this faculty visits us with remorse, *after* offences are actually committed, instead of arresting our hands by an irresistible veto before them, so as to save us from the perpetration altogether. The problem is solved by the principle, that happiness consists in the activity of our faculties, and that the arrangement of punishment after the offence is far more conducive to activity than the opposite. For example; if we desired to enjoy the highest gratification of Locality, Form, Colouring, Ideality, and Wonder, in exploring a new country, replete with the most exquisite beauties of scenery and most captivating natural productions, and if we found among these, precipices that gratified Ideality in the highest degree, but which endangered life when we advanced so near as to fall over them, and neglected the law of gravitation, whether would it be most bountiful for Providence to send an invisible attendant with us, who, whenever we were about to approach the brink, should interpose a barrier, and fairly cut short our advance, without requiring us to bestow one thought upon the subject, and without our knowing when to expect it and when not,—or to leave all open, but to confer on us, as he has done, eyes fitted to see the precipice, faculties to comprehend the law of gravitation, Cautiousness to make us fear the infringement of it, and then to leave us to enjoy the scene in perfect safety if we used these powers, but to fall over and suffer pain by bruises and death if we neglected to exercise them? It is obvious that the latter arrangement would give far more scope to our various powers; and if active faculties are the sources of pleasure, as will be shown in the next section, then it would contribute more to our enjoyment than the other. Now, Conscientiousness punishing after the fact, is analogous in the moral world, to this arrangement, in the physical. If Intellect, Benevolence, Veneration, and Conscientiousness, do their parts, they will give distinct intimations of disapprobation before commission of the offence, just as Cautiousness will give intimations of danger at sight of the cliff; but if these are disregarded, and we fall over the moral precipice, remorse follows as the punishment, just as pain is the chastisement for tumbling over the physical brink. The object of both institutions is to permit and encourage the most vigorous and unrestrained exercise of our faculties, in accordance with the physical, moral, and intellectual laws of nature, and to punish us only when we transgress these limits.

FIRMNESS is bestowed,—and the other faculties of the mind are its objects. It supports and maintains their activity, and gives determination to our purposes.

The next Class of Faculties is the Intellectual.

The provisions in external nature for the gratification of the *Senses* of Hearing, Seeing, Smelling, Taste, and Touch, or Feeling, are so obvious that it is unnecessary to enlarge upon them.

INDIVIDUALITY and EVENTUALITY, or the powers of observing things that exist, and occurrences, are given, and 'all the truths which Natural Philosophy teaches, depend upon *matter of fact*, and that is learned by observation and experiment, and never could be discovered by reasoning at all.' Here, then, is ample scope for the exercise of these powers.

FORM, SIZE, WEIGHT, LOCALITY, ORDER, NUMBER, are bestowed, and the sciences of Geometry, Arithmetic, Algebra, Geography, Chemistry, Botany, Mineralogy, Zoology, Anatomy, and various others, exist, as the fields of their exercise. The first three sciences are almost the entire products of these faculties; the others result chiefly from them, when applied on external objects.

COLOURING, } are given, { and these, aided by Constructiveness, Form, Locality, Ideality, and other faculties, find scope in Painting, Sculpture, Poetry, and the other fine arts.
TIME,
TUNE,

LANGUAGE is given,—and our faculties inspire us with lively emotions and ideas, which we desire to communicate by its means to other individuals.

COMPARISON, } exist, { and these faculties, aided by Individuality, Form, Size, Weight, and others already enumerated, find ample gratification in Natural Philosophy, in Moral, Political, and Intellectual Science, and their different branches.
CAUSALITY,
WIT,

IMITATION is bestowed,—and everywhere man is surrounded by beings and objects whose actions and appearances it may benefit him to copy.

SECTION VI.

ON THE SOURCES OF HUMAN HAPPINESS, AND THE CONDITIONS REQUISITE FOR MAINTAINING IT.

HAVING now given a rapid sketch of the Constitution of Man, and its relations to external objects, we are prepared to inquire into the sources of his happiness, and the conditions requisite for maintaining it.

The *first* and most obvious circumstance which attracts attention, is, that all enjoyment must necessarily arise from *activity* of the various systems of which the human constitution is composed. The bones, muscles, nerves, digestive and respiratory organs, furnish pleasing sensations, directly or indirectly, when exercised in conformity with their nature; and the external senses, and internal faculties, when excited, supply the whole remaining perceptions and emotions, which, when combined, constitute life and rational existence. If these were habitually buried in sleep, or constitutionally inactive, life, to all purposes of enjoyment, might as well be extinct; for existence would be reduced to mere vegetation, without Consciousness.

If, then, Wisdom and Benevolence have been employed in constituting Man, we may expect the arrangements of creation, in regard to him, to be calculated *as a leading object to excite* his various powers, corporeal and mental, *to activity.* This, accordingly, appears to me to be the case; and the fact may be illustrated by a few examples. A certain portion of nervous and muscular energy is infused by nature into the human body every twenty-four hours, and it is delightful to expend this vigour. To provide for its expenditure, the stomach has been constituted so as to require regularly returning supplies of food, which can be obtained only by nervous and muscular exertion; the body has been created destitute of covering, yet standing in need of protection from the elements of Heaven; but this can be easily provided by moderate expenditure of corporeal strength. It is delightful to repair exhausted nervous and muscular energy, by wholesome aliment; and the digestive organs have been so constituted, as to perform their functions by successive stages, and to afford us frequent opportunities of enjoying the pleasures of eating. In these arrangements, the design of supporting the various systems of the body in activity, for the enjoyment of the individual, is abundantly obvious. A late writer justly remarks, that ' a person of feeble texture and indolent habits has the bone smooth, thin, and light; but nature, solicitous for our safety, in a manner which we could not anticipate, combines with the powerful muscular frame a dense and perfect texture of bone, where every spine and tubercle is completely developed.' ' As the structure of the parts is originally perfected by the action of the vessels, the function or operation of the part is made the stimulus to those vessels. The cuticle on the hand wears away like a glove; but the pressure stimulates the living surface to force successive layers of skin under that which is wearing, or, as anatomists call it, desquamating; by which they mean, that the cuticle does not change at once, but comes off in squamæ or scales.'

Directing our attention to the Mind, we discover that Individuality, and the other Perceptive Faculties, desire, as *their* means of enjoyment, to know existence, and to become acquainted with the qualities of external objects; while the Reflecting Faculties desire to know their dependences and relations. 'There is something,' says an eloquent writer, 'positively agreeable to all men, to all, at least whose nature is not most grovelling and base, in gaining knowledge for its own sake. When you see anything for the first time, you at once derive some gratification from the sight being new; your attention is awakened, and you desire to know more about it. If it is a piece of workmanship, as an instrument, a machine of any kind, you wish to know how it is made; how it works; and what use it is of. If it is an animal, you desire to know where it comes from; how it lives; and what are its dispositions, and generally, its nature and habits. This desire is felt, too, without at all considering that the machine or the animal may ever be of the least use to yourself practically; for, in all probability, you may never see them again. But you feel a curiosity to learn all about them, *because they are new and unknown to you.* You, accordingly make inquiries; you *feel a gratification* in getting answers to your questions, that is, *in receiving information,* and in knowing more,—in being better informed than you were before. If you ever happen again to see the same instrument or animal, you find it agreeable to recollect having seen it before, and to think that you know something about it. If you see another instrument or animal, in some respects like it, but differing in other particulars, you find it pleasing to *compare them together,* and to note in what they agree, and in what they differ. Now, all this kind of gratification is of a pure and disinterested nature, and has no reference to any of the common purposes of life; yet it is a pleasure—an enjoyment. You are nothing the richer for it; you do not gratify your palate, or any other bodily appetite; and yet it is so pleasing that you would give something out of your pocket to obtain it, and would forego some bodily enjoyment for its sake. The pleasure derived from science is exactly of the like nature, or rather it is the very same.'* This is a correct and forcible exposition of the pleasures attending the active exercise of our intellectual faculties.

Supposing the human faculties to have received their present constitution, two arrangements may be fancied as instituted for the gratification of these powers. 1st. Infusing into them at birth *intuitive knowledge* of every object which they are fitted ever to comprehend; or, 2*dly.* Constituting them only as *capacities* for gaining knowledge by exercise and application, and surrounding them with objects bearing such relations towards them, that, when observed and attended to, they shall afford them high gratification; and, when unobserved and neglected, they shall occasion them uneasiness and pain; and the question occurs, Which mode would be most conducive to enjoyment? The general opinion will be in favour of the first; but the second appears to me to be preferable. If the first meal we had eaten had forever prevented the recurrence of hunger, it is obvious that all the pleasures of satisfying a healthy appetite would have been then at an end; so that this apparent bounty would have greatly abridged our enjoyment. In like manner, if, our faculties being constituted as at present, intuitive knowledge had been communicated to us, so that, when an hour old, we should have been thoroughly acquainted with every object, quality, and relation that we could ever comprehend, all provision for the sustained activity of many of our faculties would have been

---

*Objects, Advantages, and Pleasures of Science, page 1.

done away with. When wealth is acquired, the miser's pleasure in it is diminished. He grasps after *more* with increasing avidity. He is supposed irrational in doing so; but he obeys the instinct of his nature. What he possesses, no longer satisfies Acquisitiveness; it is like food in the stomach, which gave pleasure in eating, and would give pain were it withdrawn, but which, when there, is attended with little positive sensation. The Miser's pleasure arises from the *active state* of Acquisitiveness, and only the pursuit and obtaining of *new treasures* can *maintain this state*. The same law is exemplified in the case of Love of Approbation. The gratification which it affords depends on its *active state*, and hence the necessity for *new incense*, and *higher mounting* in the scale of ambition, is constantly experienced by its victims. NAPOLEON, in exile, said 'Let us live upon the past:' but he found this impossible; his predominating desires originated in Ambition and Self-esteem; and the past did not stimulate these powers, or maintain them in constant activity. In like manner, no musician, artist, poet, or philosopher, would reckon himself happy, however extensive his attainments, if informed, Now you must stop, and live upon the past; and the reason is still the same. New ideas, and new emotions, best excite and maintain in activity the faculties of the mind, and activity is essential to enjoyment. If these views be correct, the consequences of imbuing the mind with intuitive knowledge, would not have been unquestionably beneficial. The limits of our acquirements would have been reached; our first step would have been our last: every object would have become old and familiar; Hope would have had no object of expectation; Cautiousness no object of fear; Wonder no gratification in novelty; monotony, insipidity, and mental satiety, would apparently have been the lot of man.

According to the view now advanced, creation, in its present form, is more wisely and benevolently adapted to our constitution than if intuitive instruction had been showered on the mind at birth. By the actual arrangement, numerous noble faculties are bestowed; their objects are presented to them; these objects are naturally endowed with qualities fitted to benefit and delight us, when their uses and proper applications are discovered, and to injure and punish us for our ignorance, when their properties are misunderstood or misapplied; but we are left to find out all these qualities and relations by the exercise of the faculties themselves. In this manner, provision is made for ceaseless activity of the mental powers, and this constitutes the greatest delight. Wheat, for instance, is produced by the earth, and admirably adapted to the nutrition of the body; but it may be rendered more grateful to the organ of taste, more salubrious to the stomach, and more stimulating to the nervous and muscular systems, by being stripped of its external skin, ground into flour, and baked by fire into bread. Now, the Creator obviously pre-arranged all these relations, when he endowed wheat with its properties, and the human body with its qualities and functions. In withholding congenital and intuitive knowledge of these qualities and mutual relations, but in bestowing faculties of Individuality, Form, Colouring, Weight, Constructiveness, &c. fitted to find them out; in rendering the exercise of these faculties agreeable; and in leaving man, in this condition, to proceed for himself,—he appears to me to have conferred on him the highest boon. The earth produces also hemlock and foxglove; and, by the organic law, those substances, if taken in certain moderate quantities, remove diseases; if in excess, they occasion death: but, again, man's observing faculties are fitted, when applied under the guidance of Cautiousness and Reflection, to make this discovery; and he is left to make it in this way, or suffer the consequences of neglect.

Further, water, when elevated in temperature, becomes steam; and steam expands with prodigious power; this power, confined by muscular energy, exerted on metal, and directed by intellect, is capable of being converted into the steam-engine, the most efficient, yet humble servant of man. All this was clearly pre-arranged by the Creator; and man's faculties were adapted to it; but still we see him left to observe and discover the qualities and relations of water for himself. This duty, however, must be acknowledged as benevolently imposed, the moment we discover that the Creator has made the very exercise of the faculties pleasurable, and arranged external qualities and relations so beneficially, that, when known, they carry a double reward in adding by their positive influence to human gratification.

The Knowing Faculties, as we have seen, observe the mere external qualities of bodies, and their simpler relations. The Reflecting Faculties observe relations also; but of a higher order. The former, for example, discover that the soil is clay or gravel; that it is tough or friable; that it is wet, and that excess of water impedes vegetation; that in one season the crop is large, and in the next deficient. The reflecting faculties take cognizance of the *causes* of these phenomena. They discover the *means* by which wet soil may be rendered dry; clay may be pulverized; light soil may be invigorated; and all of them made more productive; also the relationship of particular soils to particular kinds of grain. The inhabitants of a country who exert their knowing faculties of their soil, their reflecting faculties in discovering its capabilities and relations to water, lime, manures, and the various species of grain, and who put forth their muscular and nervous energies in accordance with the dictates of these powers, receive a rich reward in a climate improved in salubrity, in an abundant supply of food, besides much positive enjoyment attending the exercise of the powers themselves. Those communities, on the other hand, who neglect to use their mental faculties and muscular and nervous energies, are punished by ague, fever, rheumatism, and a variety of painful affections, arising from damp air; are stinted in food; and, in wet seasons, are brought to the very brink of starvation by total failure of their crops. This punishment is a benevolent admonition from the Creator, that they are neglecting a great duty, and omitting to enjoy a great pleasure; and it will cease as soon as they have fairly redeemed the blessings lost by their negligence, and obeyed the laws of their being.

The winds and waves appear, at first sight, to present insurmountable obstacles to man leaving the island or continent on which he happens to be born, and to his holding intercourse with his fellows in distant climes : But, by observing the relations of water to timber, he is able to construct a ship; by observing the influence of the wind on a physical body placed in a fluid medium, he discovers the use of sails; and, finally, by the application of his faculties, he has found out the expansive quality of steam, and traced its relations until he has produced a machine that enables him almost to set the roaring tempest at defiance, and to sail straight to the stormy north, although its loudest and its fiercest blasts oppose. In these instances, we perceive external nature admirably adapted to support the mental faculties in habitual activity, and to reward us for the exercise of them.

It is objected to this argument, that it involves an inconsistency. Ignorance, it is said, of the natural laws, is necessary to happiness, in order that the faculties may obtain exercise in discovering them;—nevertheless, happiness is impossible till these laws shall have been discovered and obeyed. Here, then, it is said, ignorance is represented as at once *essential* to, and *incompatible* with enjoyment. The same objection, however, applies to the case of the bee. Gathering honey is necessary to its enjoyment; yet it cannot subsist and be happy till it has gathered honey, and therefore that act is both essential to, and incompatible with its gratification. The fallacy lies in losing sight of the natural constitution both of the bee and of man. While the bee possesses instinctive tendencies to roam about the fields and flowery meadows, and to exert its energies in labour, it is obviously beneficial to it to be furnished with motives and opportunities for doing so; and so it is with man to obtain scope for his bodily and mental powers. Now, gathering knowledge is to the mind of man what gathering honey is to the bee. Apparently with the view of effectually prompting the bee to seek this pleasure, honey is made essential to its subsistence. In like manner, and probably with a similar design, knowledge is made indispensable to human enjoyment. Communicating intuitive knowledge of the natural laws to man, *while his present constitution continues*, would be the exact parallel of gorging the bee with honey in midsummer, when its energies are at their heignt. When the bee has completed its store, winter benumbs its powers, which resume their vigor only when its stock is exhausted, and spring returns to afford them scope. No torpor resembling that of winter seals up the faculties of the human race; but their ceaseless activity is amply provided for. *First*, The laws of nature, compared with the mind of any individual, are of boundless extent, so that every one may learn something new to the end of the longest life. *Secondly*, By the actual constitution of man, he must make use of his acquirements habitually, otherwise he will lose them. *Thirdly*, Every individual of the race is born in utter ignorance, and starts from zero in the scale of knowledge, so that he has the laws to learn for himself.

These circumstances remove the apparent inconsistency. If man had possessed intuitive knowledge of all nature, he could have had no scope for exercising his faculties in *acquiring* knowledge, in *preserving* it, or in *communicating* it. The infant would have been as wise as the most revered sage, and forgetfulness would have been necessarily excluded.

Those who object to these views, imagine that after the human race has acquired knowledge of all the natural laws, if such a result be possible, they *will be in the same condition as if they had been created with intuitive knowledge;* but this does not follow. Although the *race* should acquire the knowledge supposed, it is not an inevitable consequence that *each individual* will necessarily enjoy it all; which, however, would follow from intuition. The entire soil of Britain belongs to the landed proprietors as a class; but each does not possess it *all;* and hence every one has scope for adding to his territories; with this advantage, however, in favour of knowledge, that the acquisitions of one do not impoverish another. Further, although the race should have learned all the natural laws, their children would not intuitively inherit their ideas, and hence the activity of every one, as he appears on the stage, would be provided for; whereas, by intuition, every child would be as wise as his grandfather, and parental protection, filial piety, and all the delights that spring from difference in knowledge between youth and age, would be excluded. 3d, *Using* of acquirements, is, by the actual state of man, essential to the preservation as well as the enjoyment of them. By intuition all knowledge would be habitually present to the mind without effort or consideration. On the whole, therefore, it appears that man's nature being what it is, the arrangement by which he is endowed with powers to acquire knowledge, but left to find it out for himself, is both wise and benevolent.

It has been asked, 'But is there no pleasure in science but that of discovery? Is there none in using the knowledge we have attained? Is there no pleasure in playing at chess after we know the moves?' In answer, I observe, that if we know beforehand all the moves that our antagonist intends to make and all our own, which must be the case if we know *everything* by intuition, we shall have no pleasure. The pleasure really consists in discovering the intentions of our antagonist, and in calculating the effects of our own play; a certain degree of ignorance of both of which is indispensable to gratification. In like manner, it is agreeable first to discover the natural laws, and then to study ' the moves' that we ought to make, in consequence of knowing them. So much, then, for the *sources* of human happiness.

In the *second* place, To reap enjoyment in the *greatest quantity*, and to maintain it *most permanently*, the faculties must be gratified *harmoniously:* In other words, if, among the various powers, the *supremacy* belongs to the moral sentiments, then the aim of our habitual conduct must be the attainment of objects suited to gratify them. For example, in pursuing wealth or fame as the leading object of existence, full gratification is not afforded to Benevolence, Veneration, and Conscientiousness, and, consequently, complete satisfaction cannot be enjoyed; whereas, by seeking knowledge, and dedicating life to the welfare of mankind and obedience to God, in our several vocations, these faculties will be gratified, and wealth, fame, health, and other advantages, will flow in their train, so that the whole mind will rejoice, and its delights will remain permanent as long as the conduct continues to be in accordance with the supremacy of the moral powers and the laws of external creation.

Thirdly, To place human happiness on a secure basis, the laws of external creation themselves must accord with the dictates of the moral sentiments, and intellect must be fitted to discover the nature and relations of both, and to direct the conduct in coincidence with them.

Much has been written about the extent of human ignorance; but we should discriminate between absolute incapacity to know, and mere want of information arising from not having used this capacity to its full extent. In regard to the first, or our capacity to know, it appears probable that, in this world, we shall never know the essence, beginning, or end of things; because these are points which we have no faculties calculated to reach. But the same Creator who made the external world constituted our faculties, and if we have sufficient data for inferring that His intention is, that we shall enjoy existence here while preparing for the ulterior ends of our being; and if it be true that we can be happy here only by becoming acquainted with the qualities and modes of action of our own minds and bodies, with the qualities and modes of action of external objects, and with the relations established between them; in short, by becoming thoroughly conversant with those natural laws, which, when observed, are prearranged to contribute to our enjoyment, and which, when violated, visit us with suffering, we may safely conclude that our mental capacities are wisely adapted to the attainment of these objects, whenever we shall do our own duty in bringing them to their highest condition of perfection, and in applying them in the best manner.

If we advert for a moment to what we already know, we shall see that this conclusion is supported by high probabilities. Before the mariner's compass and astronomy were discovered, nothing would seem more utterly beyond the reach of the human faculties than traversing the enormous Atlantic or Pacific Oceans; but the moment these discoveries were made, how simple did this feat appear, and how completely within the scope of human ability! But it became so, not by any addition to man's mental capacities, nor by any change in the physical world; but by the easy process of applying Individuality, and the other knowing faculties, to observe, Causality to reflect, and Constructiveness to build; in short, to perform their natural functions. Who that, forty years ago, regarded the small-pox as a scourge, devastating Europe, Asia, Africa, and America, would not have despaired of the human faculties ever discovering an antidote against it? and yet we have lived to see this end accomplished by a simple exercise of Individuality and reflection, in observing the effects of, and applying vaccine inoculation. Nothing appears more completely beyond the reach of the human intellect, than the cause of volcanoes and earthquakes; and yet some approach towards its discovery has recently been made.*

Sir ISAAC NEWTON observed, that all bodies which refracted the rays of light were combustible, except one, the diamond, which he found to possess this quality, but which he was not able by any powers he possessed, to burn. He did not conclude, however, from this, that the diamond was an exception to the uniformity of nature. He inferred, that, as the same Creator made the refracting bodies which he was able to consume and the diamond, and proceeded by uniform laws, the diamond would, in all probability, be found to be combustible, and that the reason of its resisting his power, was ignorance on his part of the proper way to produce its conflagration. A century afterwards, chemists made the diamond blaze with as much vivacity as Sir Isaac Newton had done a wax candle. Let us proceed, then, on an analogous principle. If the intention of our Creator was, that we should enjoy existence while in this world, then He knew what was necessary to enable us to do so; and He will not be found to have failed in conferring on us powers fitted to accomplish His design, provided we do our duty in developing and applying them. The great motive to exertion is the conviction, that increased knowledge will furnish us with increased means of doing good,—with new proofs of benevolence and wisdom in the Great Architect of the Universe.

The human race may be regarded as only in the beginning of its existence. The art of printing is an invention comparatively but of yesterday, and no imagination can yet conceive the effects which it is destined to produce. Phrenology was wanting to give it full efficacy, especially

---

* *Vide* Codier, in Edin. New Phil. Journ. No. VIII. p. 273.

in *moral science*, in which little progress has been made for centuries. Now that this desideratum is supplied, may we not hope that the march of improvement will proceed in a rapidly accelerating ratio?

SECTION VII.

APPLICATION OF THE NATURAL LAWS TO THE PRACTICAL ARRANGEMENTS OF LIFE.

IF a system of living and occupation were to be framed for human beings, founded on the exposition of their nature, which I have now given, it would be something like this.

1*st*. So many hours a day would require to be dedicated by every individual in health, to the exercise of his nervous and muscular systems, in labour calculated to give scope to these functions. The reward of obeying this requisite of his nature would be health, and a joyous animal existence; the punishment of neglect is disease, low spirits, and death.

2*dly*. So many hours a day should be spent in the sedulous employment of the knowing and reflecting faculties; in studying the qualities of external objects, and their relations; also the nature of all animated beings, and their relations; not with the view of accumulating mere abstract and barren knowledge, but of enjoying the positive pleasure of mental activity, and of turning every discovery to account, as a means of increasing happiness, or alleviating misery. The leading object should always be to find out the relationship of every object to our own nature, organic, animal, moral, and intellectual, and to keep that relationship habitually in mind, so as to render our acquirements directly gratifying to our various faculties. The reward of this conduct would be an incalculably great increase of properties of external objects, together with a great accession of power in reaping ulterior advantages, and in avoiding disagreeable affections.

3*dly.* So many hours a day ought to be devoted to the cultivation and gratification of our moral sentiments; that is to say, in exercising these in harmony with intellect, and especially in acquiring the habit of admiring, loving, and yielding obedience to the Creator and his institutions. This last object is of vast importance. Intellect is barren of practical fruit, however rich it may be in knowledge, until it is fired and prompted to act by moral sentiment. In my view, knowledge by itself is comparatively worthless and impotent, compared with what it becomes when vivified by elevated emotions. It is not enough that Intellect is informed; the moral faculties must simultaneously co-operate; yielding obedience to the precepts which the intellect recognises to be true. One way of cultivating the sentiments would be for men to meet and act together, on the fixed principles which I am now endeavouring to unfold, and to exercise on each other in mutual instruction, and in united adoration of the great and glorious Creator, the several faculties of Benevolence, Veneration, Hope, Ideality, Wonder, and Justice. The reward of acting in this manner would be a communication of direct and intense pleasure to each other; for I refer to every individual who has ever had the good fortune to pass a day or an hour with a really benevolent, pious, honest, and intellectual man, whose soul swelled with adoration of his Creator, whose intellect was replenished with knowledge of his works, and whose whole mind was instinct with sympathy for human happiness, whether such a day did not afford him the most pure, elevated, and lasting gratification he ever enjoyed. Such an exercise, besides, would invigorate the whole moral and intellectual powers, and fit them to discover and obey the divine institutions.

pleasure, in the very act of acquiring knowledge of the real

Phrenology is highly conducive to this enjoyment of our moral and intellectual nature. No faculty is bad, but, on the contrary each, when properly gratified, is a fountain of pleasure; in short, man possesses no feeling, of the legitimate exercise of which an enlightened and ingenuous mind need be ashamed. A party of thorough practical phrenologists, therefore, meets in the perfect knowledge of each other's qualities; they respect these as the gifts of the Creator, and their great object is to derive the utmost pleasure from their legitimate use, and to avoid every approximation to abuse of them. The distinctions of country and temperament are broken down by unity of principle; the chilling restraints of Cautiousness, Self-esteem, Secretiveness, and Love of Approbation, which stand as barriers of eternal ice between human beings in the ordinary intercourse of society, are gently removed; the directing sway is committed to Benevolence, Veneration, Conscientiousness, and Intellect; and then the higher principles of the mind operate with a delightful vivacity unknown to persons unacquainted with the qualities of human nature.

Intellect also ought to be regularly exercised in arts, science, philosophy, and observation.

I have said nothing of dedicating hours to the direct gratification of the animal powers; not that they should not be exercised, but that full scope for their activity will be included in the employments already mentioned. In muscular exercises, Combativeness, Destructiveness, Constructiveness, Acquisitiveness, Self-esteem, and Love of Approbation, may all be gratified. In contending with and surmounting physical and moral difficulties, Combativeness and Destructiveness obtain vent; in working at a mechanical employment, requiring the exertion of strength, these two faculties, and also Constructiveness and Acquisitiveness, will be exercised; in emulation who shall accomplish most good, Self-esteem and Love of Approbation will obtain scope. In the exercise of the moral faculties, several of these and others of the animal propensities, are employed; Amativeness, Philoprogenitiveness, and Adhesiveness, for example, acting under the guidance of Benevolence, Veneration, Conscientiousness, Ideality, and Intellect receive direct enjoyment in the domestic circle. From proper direction also, and from the superior delicacy and refinement imparted to them by the higher powers, they do not infringe the moral law, and leave no sting or repentance in the mind.

Finally, a certain portion of time would require to be dedicated to taking of food and sleep.

All systems hitherto practised have been deficient in providing for one or more of these branches of enjoyment. In the community at Orbiston, formed on Mr. OWEN's principles, music, dancing, and theatrical entertainments were provided; but the people soon tired of these. They had not corresponding moral and intellectual instruction. The novelty excited them, but there was nothing substantial behind. In common society, very little either of rational instruction or amusement is provided. The neglect of innocent amusement is a great error.

If there be truth in these views, they will afford answers to two important questions, that have puzzled philosophers in regard to the progress of human improvement. The first is, why should man have existed so long, and made so small an advance in the road to happiness?* If I am right in the fundamental proposition, that activity in the faculties is synonymous with enjoyment of existence,—it follows that it would have been less wise and benevolent towards man, constituted as he is, to have communicated to him intuitively perfect knowledge, thereby leaving his mental powers with diminished motives to activity, than to bestow on him faculties endowed with high susceptibility of action,

---

* In offering a solution of this problem, I do not inquire why man has received his present constitution.

and to surround him with scenes, objects, circumstances, and relations, calculated to maintain them in ceaseless excitement; although this latter arrangement necessarily subjects him to suffering while ignorant, and renders his first ascent in the scale of improvement difficult and slow. It is interesting to observe, that, according to this view, although the first pair of the human race had been created with powerful and well balanced faculties, but of the same nature as at present; if they were not also intuitively inspired with knowledge of the whole creation, and its relations, their first movements as *individuals* would have been *retrograde*; that is, as *individuals*, they would, through pure want of information, have infringed many natural laws, and suffered evil; while, as *parts of the race*, they would have been decidedly *advancing;* for every pang they suffered would have led them to a new step in knowledge, and prompted them to advance towards a much higher condition than that which they at first occupied. According to the hypothesis now presented, not only is man really benefited by the arrangement which leaves him to discover the natural laws for himself, although during the period of his ignorance, he suffers much evil from unacquaintance with them; but *his progress* towards knowledge and happiness must from the very extent of his experience, *be actually greater* than can at present be conceived. Its extent will become more obvious, and his experience itself more valuable, after he has obtained a view of the real theory of his constitution. He will find that past miseries have at least exhausted countless errors, and he will know how to avoid thousands of paths that lead to pain; in short, he will then discover that errors in conduct resemble errors in philosophy, in this, that they give additional importance and practicability to truth, by the demonstration which they afford of the evils attending departures from its dictates. The grand sources of human suffering at present arise from bodily disease and mental distress, and, in the next chapter, these will be traced to infringement, through ignorance or otherwise, of physical, organic, moral, or intellectual laws, which, when expounded, appear in themselves calculated to promote the happiness of the race. It may be supposed that, according to this view, as knowledge accumulates, enjoyment will decrease; but ample provision is made against this event, by withholding intuition from each generation as it appears on the stage; each successive age must acquire knowledge for itself; and, provided ideas are new, and suited to the faculties, the pleasure of acquiring them from instructers, is only second to that of discovering them for ourselves; and, probably countless ages may elapse before *all* the facts and relations of nature shall have been explored, and the possibility of discovery exhausted. If the universe be infinite, knowledge can never be complete.

The second question is, Has man really advanced in happiness, in proportion to his increase in knowledge? We are apt to entertain erroneous notions of the pleasures enjoyed by past ages. Fabulists have represented them as peaceful, innocent, and gay; but if we look narrowly at the condition of the savage and barbarian of the present day, and recollect that these are the states of all individuals previous to the acquisition of knowledge, we shall not much or long regret the pretended diminution of enjoyment by civilization. Phrenology renders the superiority of the latter condition certain, by showing it to be a law of nature, that, until the intellect is extensively informed, and the moral sentiments assiduously exercised, the animal propensities bear the predominat sway; and that wherever they are supreme, misery is an inevitable concomitant. Indeed, the answer to the objection that happiness has not increased with knowledge, appears to me to be found in the fact, that until phrenology was discovered, the nature of man was not scientifically known; and in consequence, that not one of his institutions, civil or domestic, was correctly founded on the principle of the supremacy of the moral sentiments, or in accordance with the other laws of his constitution. Owing to the same cause, also, much of his knowledge has necessarily remained partial, and inapplicable to use; but after this science shall have been appreciated and applied, clouds of darkness, accumulated through long ages that are past, may be expected to roll away, as if touched by the rays of the meridian sun, and with them many of the miseries that attend total ignorance or imperfect information.*

CHAPTER III.

TO WHAT EXTENT ARE THE MISERIES OF MANKIND REFERABLE TO INFRINGEMENTS OF THE LAWS OF NATURE?

In the present chapter, I propose to inquire into some of the evils that have afflicted the human race; also whether they have proceeded from abuses of institutions benevolent and wise in themselves, and calculated, when observed, to promote the happiness of man, or from a defective or vicious constitution of nature, which he can neither remedy nor improve.

SECTION I.—CALAMITIES ARISING FROM INFRINGEMENTS OF THE PHYSICAL LAWS.

The proper way of viewing the Creator's institutions, is to look, first, to their uses, and to the advantages that flow

---

* Readers who are strangers to phrenology, and the evidence on which it rests, may regard the observations in the text as extravagant and enthusiastic; but I respectfully remind them, that, while they judge in comparative ignorance, it has been my endeavour to subject it to the severest scrutiny. Having found its proofs irrefragable, and being convinced of its importance, I solicit their indulgence in speaking of it as it appears to my own mind.

from observance of them; and, secondly, to their abuses, and the evils consequent thereon.

In Chapter II., some of the benefits conferred on man, by the law of gravitation, are enumerated; and I may here advert to the evils originating from that law, when human conduct is in opposition to it. For example, men are liable to fall from horses, carriages, stairs, precipices, roofs, chimneys, ladders, masts, to slip in the street, &c., by which accidents life is frequently altogether extinguished, or rendered miserable from lameness and pain; and the question arises, Is human nature provided with any means of protection against these evils, at all equal to their frequency and extent.

The lower animals are equally subject to this law; and the Creator has bestowed on them external senses, nerves, muscles, bones, an instinctive sense of equilibrium, the sense of danger, or cautiousness, and other faculties, to place them in accordance with it. These appear to afford sufficient protection to animals placed in all ordinary circumstances; for we very rarely discover any of them, in their natural condition, killed or mutilated by accidents referable to gravitation. Where their mode of life exposes them to extraordinary danger from this law, they are provided with additional securities. The monkey, which climbs trees, enjoys great muscular energy in its legs, claws, and tail, far surpassing, in proportion to its gravitating tendency, or its bulk and weight, what is bestowed on the legs and arms of man; so that, by means of them, it springs from branch to branch, in nearly complete security against the law in question. The goat, which browses on the brinks of precipices, has received a hoof and legs, that give precision and stability to its steps. Birds, which are destined to sleep on branches of trees, are provided with a muscle passing over the joints of each leg, and stretching down to the foot, which, being pressed by their weight, produces a proportionate contraction of their claws, so as to make them cling the faster, the greater their liability to fall. The fly, which walks and sleeps on perpendicular walls, and the ceilings of rooms, has a hollow in its foot, from which it expels the air, and the pressure of the atmosphere on the outside of the foot holds it fast to the object on which the inside is placed. The sea-horse, which is destined to climb up the sides of ice-hills, is provided with a similar apparatus. The camel, whose native region is the sandy deserts of the torrid zone, has broad spreading hooves to support it on the loose soil. Fishes are furnished with air bladders, by dilating and contracting of which they can accommodate themselves with perfect precision to the law of gravitation.

In these instances, the lower animals, under the sole guidance of their instincts, appear to be placed admirably in harmony with gravitation, and guaranteed against its infringement. Is Man, then, less an object of love with the Creator? Is he alone left exposed to the evils that spring inevitably from its neglect? His means of protection are different, but when understood and applied, they will probably be found not less complete. Man, as well as the lower animals, has received bones, muscles, nerves, an instinct of equilibrium,* and organs of Cautiousness; but not in equal perfection, in proportion to his figure, size, and weight, with those bestowed on them :—The difference, however, is far more than compensated by other organs, particularly those of Constructiveness and Reflection, in which he greatly surpasses them. Keeping in view that the external world, in regard to man, is arranged on the principle of supremacy in moral sentiments and intellect, we shall probably find, that the calamities suffered by him from the law of gravitation, are referable to predominance of the animal propensities, or to neglect of proper exercise of his intellectual powers. For example, when coaches

---

* *Vide* Essay on Weight, Phren. Journ. vol. ii. p. 412.

break down, ships sink, men fall from ladders, &c., how generally may the cause be traced to decay in the vehicle, the vessel, or ladder, which a predominating Acquisitiveness alone prevented from being repaired; or when men fall from houses, scaffolds, or slip on the street, &c., how frequently should we find their muscular, nervous, and mental energies, impaired by preceding debaucheries; in other words, by predominance of the animal faculties, which, for the time, diminished their natural means of accommodating themselves to the law from which they suffer. Or, again, the slater, in using a ladder, assists himself by Constructiveness and Reflection; but, in walking along the ridge of a house, or standing on a chimney, he takes no aid from these faculties; he trusts to the mere instinctive power of equilibrium, in which he is inferior to the lower animals, and, in so doing, clearly violates the law of his nature, that requires him to use reflection, where instinct is deficient. Causality and Constructiveness could invent means by which, if he slipped from a roof or chimney, his fall might be arrested. A small chain, for instance, attached by one end to a girdle round his body, and the other end fastened by a hook and eye to the roof, might leave him at liberty to move about, and break his fall, in case he slipped. How frequently, too, do these accidents happen, after disturbance of the faculties and corporeal functions by intoxication?

The objection will probably occur, that in the gross condition in which the mental powers exist, the great body of mankind are incapable of exerting habitually that degree of moral and intellectual energy, which is indispensable to observance of the natural laws; and that, therefore, they are, in point of fact, less fortunate, than the lower animals. I admit, that, at present, this representation is to a considerable extent just; but nowhere do I perceive the human powers exercised and instructed, in a degree at all approaching to their limits. Let any person recollect of how much greater capacity for enjoyment and security from danger he has been conscious, at a particular time, when his whole mind was filled with, and excited by, some mighty interest, not only allied to, but founded in, morality and intellect, than in that languid condition which accompanies the absence of elevated and ennobling motives, and he may form some idea of what man is capable of reaching when his powers shall have been cultivated to the extent of their capacity. At the present moment, no class of society is systematically instructed in the constitution of their own minds and bodies, in the relations of these to external objects, in the nature of these objects, in the natural supremacy of the moral sentiments, in the principle that activity in the faculties is the only source of pleasure, and that the higher the powers, the more intense the delight; and, if such views be to the mind, what light is to the eyes, air to the lungs, and food to the stomach, there is no wonder that a mass of inert *mentality*, if I may use such a word, should everywhere exist around us, and that countless evils should spring from its continuance in this condition. If active moral and intellectual faculties are the natural fountains of enjoyment, and the external world is created with reference to this state; it is as obvious that misery must result from animal supremacy and intellectual torpidity, as that flame, which is constituted to burn only when supplied with oxygen, must inevitably become extinct, when exposed to carbonic acid gas. Finally, if the arrangement by which man is left to discover and obey the laws of his own nature, and of the physical world, be more conducive to activity, than intuitive knowledge, the calamities now contemplated appear to be instituted to force him to his duty; and his duty, when understood, will constitute his delight.

While, therefore, we lament the fate of individual victims to the law of gravitation, we cannot condemn that law itself. If it were suspended, to save men from the effects of negligence, not only would the proud creations of human skill totter to their base, and the human body rise from the earth, and hang midway in the air, but our highest enjoyments would be terminated, and our faculties become positively useless, by being deprived of their field of exertion. Causality, for instance, teaches that similar causes will always, *cæteris paribus*, produce similar effects; and, if the physical laws were suspended or varied, to accommodate man's negligence or folly, it is obvious that this faculty would be without an object, and that no definite course of action could be entered upon with confidence in the result. If, then, this view of the constitution of nature were kept steadily in view, the occurrence of one accident of this kind would suggest to Reflection means to prevent others.

Similar illustrations and commentaries might be given, in regard to the other physical laws to which man is subject; but the object of the present Essay being merely to evolve principles, I confine myself to gravitation, as the most obvious and best understood.

I do not mean to say, that, by the mere exercise of intellect, man may absolutely guarantee himself against all accidents; but only that the more ignorant and careless he is, the more he will suffer, and the more intelligent and vigilant, the less; and that I can perceive no limits to this rule. The law of most civilized countries recognizes this principle, and subjects owners of ships, coaches, and other vehicles, in damages arising from gross infringements of the physical laws. It is unquestionable that the enforcement of this liability has increased security in travelling in no trifling degree.

SECTION II.

ON THE EVILS THAT BEFALL MANKIND, FROM INFRINGEMENT OF THE ORGANIC LAWS.

An organzied being, I have said, is one which derives its existence from a previously existing organized being, which subsists on food, grows, attains maturity, decays and dies. Whatever the ultimate object of the Creator, in constituting organized beings, may be, it will scarcely be denied, that part of His design is, that they should enjoy their existence here; and, if so, every particular part of their system will be found conducive in its intention to this end. The first law, then, that must be obeyed, to render an organized being perfect in its kind, is, that the germ from which it springs shall be complete in all its parts, and sound in its whole constitution; the second is, that the moment it is ushered into life, and as long as it continues to live, it shall be supplied with food, light, air, and every physical aliment necessary for its support; and the third law is, that it shall duly exercise its functions. When all these laws are obeyed, the being should enjoy pleasure from its organized frame, if its Creator is benevolent; and its constitution should be so adapted to its circumstances, as to admit of obedience to them, if its Creator is wise and powerful. Is there, then, no such phenomenon on earth, as a human being existing in full possession of organic vigour, from birth till advanced age, when the organized system is fairly worn out? Numberless examples of this kind have occurred, and they show to demonstration, that the corporeal frame of man is so constituted, as to admit the *possibility* of his enjoying organic health and vigour, during the whole period of a long life. In the life of Captain Cook it is mentioned, that 'one circumstance peculiarly worthy of notice is, the perfect and uninterrupted health of the inhabitants of New Zealand. In all the visits made to their towns, where old and young, men and women, crowded about our voyagers, they never observed a single person who appeared to have any bodily complaint; nor among the numbers that were seen naked, was once perceived the slightest eruption upon the skin, or least mark which indicated that such an eruption had formerly existed. Another proof of the health of these people is the facility with which the wounds they at any time receive are healed. In the man who had been shot with the musket ball through the fleshy part of his arm, the wound seemed to be so well digested, and in so fair a way of being perfectly healed, that if Mr. Cook had not known that no application had been made to it, he declared that he should certainly have inquired, with a very interested curiosity, after the vulnerary herbs and surgical art of the country. An additional evidence of human nature's being untainted with disease in New Zealand, is the great number of old men with which it abounds. Many of them, by the loss of their hair and teeth, appeared to be very ancient, and yet none of them were decrepit. Although they were not equal to the young in muscular strength, they did not come in the least behind them with regard to cheerfulness and vivacity. Water, as far as our navigators could discover, is the universal and only liquour of the New Zealanders. It is greatly to be wished that their happiness in this respect may never be destroyed by such a connexion with the European nations, as shall introduce that fondness for spirituous liquors which had been so fatal to the Indians of North America.'—*Kippis' Life of Captain Cook.* Dublin, 1788, p. 100.

Now, as a natural law never admits of an exception; for example, as no man ever sees without eyes, or digests without a stomach, we are entitled to say, that the best condition in which an organized being has ever been found, is fairly within the capabilities of the race. A human being, vigorous and healthy from the cradle to the grave, could no more exist, unless the natural constitution of his organs permitted it, of design, than vision could exist without eyes. Health and vigour cannot result from infringement of the organic laws; for then pain and disease would be the objects of these laws, and beneficence, wisdom, and power, could never be ascribed to the Creator, who had established them. Let us hold, then, that the organized system of man, in itself—admits of the possibility of health, vigour, and organic enjoyment, during the full period of life; and proceed to inquire into the causes why these advantages are not universal.

One organic law, is, that the germ of the infant being must be complete in all its parts, and perfectly sound in its condition, as an indispensable requisite to its vigorous developement, and full enjoyment of existence. If the corn that is sown is weak, wasted, and damaged, the plants that spring from it will be feeble, and liable to speedy decay. The same law holds in the animal kingdom; and I would ask, has it hitherto been observed by man? It is notorious that it has not. Indeed, its existence has been either altogether unknown, or in a very high degree disregarded by human beings. The feeble, the sickly, the exhausted with age, and the incompletely developed, through extreme youth, marry, and, without the least compunction regarding the organization which they shall transmit to their offspring, send into the world miserable beings, the very rudiments of whose existence are tainted with disease. If we trace such conduct to its source, we shall find it to originate either in animal propensity, intellectual ignorance, or more frequently in both. The inspiring motives are generally mere sensual appetite, avarice, or ambition, operating in the absence of all just conceptions of the impending evils. The punishment of this offence is debility and pain, transmitted to the children, and reflected back in anxiety and sorrow on the parents. Still the great point to be kept in view, is, that these miseries are not legitimate consequences of *observance* of the organic laws, but the direct chastisement of their *infringement*. These laws are unbending, and admit of no exception; they must be fulfilled, or the penalties of disobedience will follow. On this subject profound ignorance reigns in society. From such observations as I have been able to make, I am convinced that the union of certain temperaments and combinations of mental organs in the parents, are highly conducive to health, talent, and morality in the offspring, and *vice versa*, and that these conditions may be discovered and taught with far greater certainty, facility, and advantage, than is generally imagined. It will be time enough to conclude that men are naturally incapable of obedience to the organic laws, after their intellects have been instructed, their moral sentiments trained to observance of the Creator's natural institutions, as at once their duty, their interest, and a grand source of their happiness; and they have continued to rebel.

A second organic law regards nutriment, which must be supplied of a suitable kind, and in due quantity. This law requires also free air, light, cleanliness, and attention to every physical arrangement by which the functions of the body may be favoured or impaired. Have mankind, then, obeyed or neglected this institution? I need scarcely answer the question. To be able to obey institutions, we must first know them. Before we can know the organic constitution of our body, we must study that constitution, and the study of the human constitution is anatomy and physiology. Before we can be acquainted with its relations to external objects, we must learn the existence and qualities of these objects, (unfolded by chemistry, natural history, and natural philosophy,) and compare them with the constitution of the body. When we have fulfilled these conditions, we shall be better able to discover the laws which the Creator has instituted in regard to our organic system. It will be said, however, that such studies are impracticable to the great bulk of mankind, and, besides, do not appear much to benefit those who pursue them. They are impracticable only while mankind prefer founding their public and private institutions on the basis of the propensities, instead of that of the sentiments. I have mentioned, that exercise of the nervous and muscular systems is required of *all* the race by the Creator's fiat, that if all, who are capable, would obey this law, a moderate extent of exertion, agreeable and salubrious in itself, would suffice to supply our wants, and to surround us with every beneficial luxury; and that a large portion of unemployed time would remain. The Creator has bestowed on us Knowing Faculties, fitted to explore the facts of these sciences, Reflecting Faculties to trace their relations, and Moral Sentiments calculated to feel interest in such investigations, and to lead us to reverence and obey the laws which they unfold; and, finally, he has made this occupation, when entered upon with the view of tracing His power and wisdom in the subjects of our studies, and of obeying His institutions, the most delightful and invigorating of all vocations. In place, then, of such a course of education being impracticable, every arrangement of the Creator appears to be prepared in direct anticipation of its actual accomplishment.

The second objection, that those who study these sciences are not more healthy and happy, as organized beings, than those who neglect them, admits also of an easy answer. Parts of these sciences are taught to a few individuals, whose main design in studying them is to apply them as means of acquiring wealth and fame; but they have nowhere been taught as connected parts of a great system of natural arrangements, fraught with the highest influences on human enjoyment; and in no instance have the intellect and sentiments been systematically directed to the natural laws, as the grand fountains of happiness and misery to the race, and trained to observe and obey them as the Creator's institutions.

A third organic law, is, that all our functions shall be duly exercised; and is this law observed by mankind? Many persons are able, from experience, to attest the severity of the punishment that follows from neglecting to exercise the nervous and muscular systems, in the lassitude, indigestion, irritability, debility, and general uneasiness that attend a sedentary and inactive life. But the penalties that attach to neglect of exercising the *brain* are much less known, and, therefore, I shall notice them more at length. How often have we heard the question asked, What is the use of education? The answer might be illustrated by explaining to the inquirer the nature and objects of the various organs of the body, such as the limbs, lungs, eyes, and then asking him if he could perceive any advantage to a being so constituted, in obtaining access to earth, air, and light. He would, at once, declare, that they were obviously of the very highest utility to him, for they were the only conceivable objects, by means of which these organs could obtain scope for action, which action we suppose him to know to be pleasure. To those, then, who know the constitution of the intellectual and moral powers of man, I need only say, that the objects introduced to the mind by education, bear the same relation to them that the physical elements of nature bear to the nerves and muscles; they afford them scope for action, and yield them delight. The meaning which is commonly attached to the word *use* in such cases, is how much *money, influence,* or *consideration,* will education bring; these being the only objects of strong desire with which uncultivated minds are acquainted; and they do not perceive in what way education can greatly gratify such propensities. But the moment the mind is opened to the perception of its own constitution and to the natural laws, the great advantage of moral and intellectual cultivation, as a means of exercising the faculties, and of directing the conduct in obedience to these laws, becomes apparent.

But there is an additional benefit arising from healthy activity of brain, which is little known. The brain is the fountain of nervous energy to the whole body, and different modifications of that energy appear to take place, according to the mode in which the faculties and organs are affected. For example, when misfortune and disgrace impend over us, the organs of Cautiousness, Self-esteem, Love of Approbation, &c., are painfully excited; and then they transmit an impaired or a positively noxious nervous influence to the heart, stomach, intestines, and thence to the rest of the body; the pulse becomes feeble and irregular, digestion is deranged, and the whole corporeal frame wastes. When, on the other hand, the cerebral organs are agreeably affected, a benign and vivifying nervous influence pervades the frame, and all the functions of the body are performed with more pleasure and completeness. Now, it is a law, that the quantum of nervous energy increases with the number of cerebral organs roused to activity. In the retreat of the French from Moscow, for example, when no enemy was near, the soldiers became depressed in courage, and enfeebled in body, they nearly sunk to the earth through exhaustion and cold; but no sooner did the fire of the Russian guns sound in their ears, or the gleam of their bayonets flash in their eyes, than new life seemed to pervade them. They wielded powerfully the arms, which a few moments before, they could scarcely carry or trail on the ground. No sooner, however, was the enemy repulsed, than their feebleness returned. The theory of this is, that the approach of the combat called into activity a variety of additional faculties; these sent new energy through every nerve, and while their vivacity was maintained by the external stimulus, they rendered the soldiers strong beyond their merely physical condition. Many persons have probably experienced the operation of the same principle. When sitting feeble and listless by the fire, we have heard of an accident having occurred to some beloved friend, who required our instantaneous aid, or an unexpected visitor has arrived in whom our affections were bound up, in an instant our lassitude was gone, and we moved with an alertness and animation that seemed surprising to ourselves. The cause was the same; these events roused Adhesiveness, Benevolence, Love of Approbation, Intellect, and a variety of faculties, which were previously dormant, and their influence invigorated the limbs. Dr. Sparmann, in his Voyage to the Cape, mentions, that 'there was now again a great scarcity of meat in the wagon; for which reason my Hottentots began to grumble, and reminded me that we ought not to waste so much of our time in looking after insects and plants, but give a better look out after the game. At the same time, they pointed to a neighbouring dale overrun with wood, at the upper edge of which, at the distance of about a mile and a quarter from the spot where we then were, they had seen several buffaloes. Accordingly, we went thither; but though our fatigue was lessened by our Hottentots carrying our guns for us up a hill, yet we were quite out of breath, and overcome by the sun, before we got up to it. Yet, what even now appears to me a matter of wonder is, *that as soon as we got a glimpse of the game, all this languor left us in an instant.* In fact, we each of us strove to fire before the other, so that we seemed entirely to have lost sight of all prudence and caution.'—'In the mean time, our temerity, which chiefly proceeded from hurry and ignorance, was considered by the Hottentots as a proof of spirit and intrepidity hardly to be equalled.'

It is a part of the same law that the more agreeable the mental stimulus, the more benign is the nervous influence transmitted to the body.

If we imagine a man or woman, who has received from nature a large and tolerably active brain, but who has not enjoyed the advantages of a scientific or extensive education, so as to feel an interest in moral and intellectual pursuits for their own sake, and who, from possessing wealth sufficient to remove the necessity for labour, is engaged in no profession, we shall find a perfect victim to infringement of the natural laws. The individual ignorant of these laws, will, in all probability, neglect nervous and muscular exercise, and suffer the miseries arising from impeded circulation and impaired digestion; in entire want of every object on which the energy of his brain might be expended, its stimulating influence on the body will be withheld, and the effects of muscular inactivity tenfold aggravated; all the functions will, in consequence, become enfeebled; lassitude, uneasiness, anxiety, and a thousand evils, will arise, and life, in short, will become a mere endurance of punishment for infringement of institutions, calculated, in themselves, to promote happiness and afford delight, when known and obeyed. This fate frequently overtakes uneducated females, whose early days have been occupied with business, or the cares of a family, but which occupations have ceased before old age had diminished corporeal vigour; it overtakes men also, who, uneducated, retire from active business in the prime of life. In some instances, these evils accumulate to such a degree that the brain itself gives way, its functions become deranged, and insanity is the result.

It is worthy of remark, that the more elevated the objects of our study, the higher in the scale are the mental organs which are exercised, and the higher the organs the more pure and intense is the pleasure; and hence, a vivacious and regularly supported excitement of the moral sentiments and intellect, is, by the organic law, highly favourable to health and corporeal vigour. In the fact of a living animal being able to retain life in an oven that will bake dead flesh, we see an illustration of the organic law rising above the purely physical; and, in the circumstance of the moral and intellectual organs transmitting the most favourable nervous influence to the whole bodily system, we have an example of the moral and intellectual law rising higher than the mere organic.

No person after having his intellect and sentiments imbued with a perception of, and belief in, the natural laws, as now explained, can possibly desire idleness, as a source of pleasure; nor can he possibly regard musoular exertion and mental activity, when not carried to excess, as anything else than enjoyments kindly vouchsafed to him by the benevolence of the Creator. The notion that moderate labour and mental exertion are evils, can originate only from ignorance, or from viewing the effects of over-exhaustion as the result of the natural law, and not as the punishment for infringement of it.

If, then, we sedulously inquire, in each particular instance, into the *cause* of the sickness, pain, premature death, and general derangement of the corporeal frame of man, which we see around us, and endeavour to discover whether it has originated in obedience to the physical and organic laws, or sprung from infringement of them, we shall be able to form some estimate how far bodily suffering is justly attributable to imperfections of nature, and how far to our own ignorance and neglect of divine institutions.

The foregoing principles being of much practical importance, may, with propriety, be elucidated by a few cases of actual occurrence. Two or three centuries ago, various cities in Europe were depopulated by the plague, and, in particular, London was visited by an awful mortality from this cause, in the reign of Charles the Second. The people of that age attributed this scourge to the inscrutable decrees of Providence, and some to the magnitude of the nation's moral iniquities. According to the views now presented, it must have arisen from infringement of the *organic laws*, and been intended to enforce stricter obedience to them in future. According to this view, there was nothing inscrutable in its causes or objects, which, when clearly analysed, appear to have had no direct reference to the moral condition of the people: I say *direct* reference to the moral condition of the people, because it would be easy to show, that the physical, organic, and all the other natural laws, are connected indirectly, and constituted in harmony, with the moral law; and that infringement of the one often leads to disobedience to another, and brings a double punishment on the offender. But, in the mean time, I observe that the facts recorded in history exactly correspond with the theory now propounded. The streets of London were excessively narrow, the habits of the people dirty, and no adequate provision was made for removing the filth unavoidably produced by a dense population. The great fire in that city, which happened soon after the pestilence, afforded an opportunity of remedying, in some degree, the narrowness of the streets; and the habits of increasing cleanliness abated the filth; these changes brought the people into a closer obedience to the organic laws, and no plauge has since returned. Again, till very lately, thousands of children died yearly of the small-pox, but in our day, vaccine inoculation saves ninety-nine out of a hundred, who, under the old system, would have died. The theory of its operation is not known, but we may rest assured, that it places the system more in accordance with the organic laws, than in the cases where death ensued. A gentleman, who died about ten years ago at an advanced period of life, told me, that six miles west from Edinburgh, the country was so unhealthy in his youth, that every spring the farmers and their servants were seized with fever and ague, and required regularly to undergo bleeding, and a course of medicine, to prevent attacks, or restore them from their effects. At the time, these visitations were believed to be sent by Providence, and to be inherent in the constitution of things; after, however, said my informant, an improved system of agriculture and draining was established, and vast pools of stagnant water formerly left between the ridges of the field were removed, dunghills carried to a distance from the houses, and the houses themselves made more spacious and commodious, every system of ague and marsh-fever disappeared from the district, and it became highly salubrious. In other words, as soon as the gross infringement of the organic laws was abated by a more active exertion of the muscular and intellectual powers of man, the punishment ceased. In like manner, how many calamities occurred in coalpits, in consequence of infringement of a physical law, viz. by introducing lighted candles and lamps into places filled with hydrogen gas, that had emanated from seams of coal, and which exploded, scorched, and suffocated the men and animals within its reach, until Sir Humphrey Davy discovered that the Creator had established such a relation betwixt flame, wiregauze, and hydrogen gas, that by surrounding the flame with gauze, its power of exploding hydrogen was counteracted. By the simple application of a covering of wire-gauze, put over and around the flame, it is prevented from igniting gas beyond it, and colliers are now able to carry, with safety, lighted lamps into places highly impregnated with inflammable air. I have been informed, that the accidents from explosion which still occasionally occur in coal mines, arise from neglecting to keep the lamps in perfect condition.

It is needless to multiply examples in support of the proposition, that the organized system of man, in itself, admits of a healthy existence from infancy to old age, provided its germ has been healthy, and its subsequent condition has been uniformly in harmony with the physical and organic laws; but it has been objected, that although the human faculties may perhaps be adequate to discover these laws, and to record them in books, yet they are totally incapable of retaining them in the memory, and of formally applying them in every act of life. If, it is said, we could not move a step without calculating and adjusting the body to the law of gravitation, and could never eat a meal without a formal rehearsal of the organic laws, life would become oppressed by the pedantry of knowledge, and rendered miserable by petty observances and trivial details. The answer to this is, that all our faculties are adapted by the Creator to the external world, and act *instinctively* when their objects are placed in the proper light before them. For example, in walking on a footpath in the country during day, we are not conscious, in adjusting our steps to the inequalities of the surface, of being overburdened by mental calculation. In fact, we perform this adjustment with so little trouble, that we are not aware of having made *any particular* mental or muscular effort. But, on returning at night, when we cannot see, we stumble, and discover, for the first time, how important a duty our faculties had been performing during day, without our having adverted to their labours. Now, the simple medium of light is sufficient to bring clearly before our eyes the inequalities of ground; but to make the mind equally familiar with the nature of the countless objects, and their relations, which abound in external nature, an intellectual light is necessary, which can be struck out only by exercising and applying the knowing and reflecting faculties; but the moment that light is obtained, and the qualities and relationships in question are perceived by its means, the faculties, so long as the light lasts, *will act instinctively* in adapting our conduct to the nature of the objects, just as in accommodating our movements to the unequal surface of the ground. It is no more necessary for us to go through a course of physical, botanical, and chemical reasoning, before we are able to abstain from eating hemlock, after its properties are known, than it is to go through a course of mathematical demonstration, before lifting the one foot higher than the other, in ascending a stair. At present, physical and political science, morals and religion, are not taught as parts of one connected system; nor are the relations between them and the constitution of man pointed out to the world. In consequence, theoretical knowledge and practice are often widely separated. Some of the advantages of the scientific education now recommended would be the following.

In the 1st place, the physical and organic laws, when truly discovered, appear to the mind as institutions of the Creator, wise and salutary in themselves, unbending in their operation, and universal in their application. They interest our intellectual faculties, and strongly impress our sentiments. The necessity of obeying them, comes upon us with all the authority of a mandate of God. While we confine ourselves to a mere recommendation to beware of damp, to observe temperance, or to take exercise, without explaining the *principle*, the injunction carries only the weight due to *the authority of the individual* who gives it, and is addressed to only two or three faculties. Veneration and Cautiousness, for instance, or Self-love in him who receives it. But if we are made acquainted with the elements of the physical world, and with those of our organized system,—with the uses of the different parts of the latter, and the conditions necessary to their healthy action,—with the causes of their derangement, and the pains consequent thereon: and if the obligation to attend to these conditions be enforced on our moral sentiments and intellect, then the motives to observe the physical and organic laws, as well as *the power of doing so*, will be prodigiously increased. Before we can dance well, we must not only *know the motions*, but our muscles must be trained *to execute them*. In like manner, to enable us to act on precepts, we must not only comprehend their meaning, but our intellects and sentiments must be disciplined into actual performance. Now, the very act of acquiring connected scientific information concerning the natural world, its qualities, and their relations, is to the intellect and sentiments what practical dancing is to the muscles; *it invigorates them;* and, as obedience to the natural laws must spring from them, exercise renders it more easy and delightful.

2. It is only by being taught the *principle* on which consequences depend, that we see the *invariableness* of the results of the physical and organic laws; acquire confidence in, and respect for the laws themselves; and fairly endeavour to accommodate our conduct to their operation. Dr. Johnson defines 'principle' to be 'fundamental truth;

original postulate ; first position from which others are deduced ;' and in these senses I use the word. The human faculties are instinctively active, and desire gratification; but Intellect itself must have fixed data, on which to reason, otherwise it is itself a mere impulse. The man in whom Constructiveness and weight are powerful, will naturally betake himself to constructing machinery; but, if he be ignorant of the principles of mechanical science, he will not direct his efforts to as important ends, and attain them as successfully, as if his intellect were stored with these. Principles are deduced from the *laws* of nature. A man may make music by the instinctive impulses of Time and Tune; but there are immutable laws of harmony; and, if ignorant of these, he will not perform so invariably, correctly, and in good taste as if he knew them. In every art and science, there are principles referable solely to the constitution of nature, but these admit of countless applications. A musician may produce gay, grave, solemn, or ludicrous tunes, all good of their kind, by following the laws of harmony; but he will never produce one good piece by violating them. While the inhabitants west of Edinburgh allowed the stagnant pools to deface their fields, some seasons would be more healthy than others; and, while the cause of the disease was unsuspected, this would confirm them in the notion that health and sickness were dispensed by an overruling Providence, on inscrutable principles, which they could not comprehend; but the moment the cause was known, it would be found that the most healthy seasons were those that were cold and dry, and the most sickly those that were warm and moist; and they would then perceive, that the superior salubrity of one year, and unwholesomeness of another, were clearly referable to *one principle*, and would be both more strongly prompted, and rendered morally and intellectually more capable of applying the remedy. If some intelligent friend had merely told them to drain their fields, and remove their dunghills, they would not probably have done it; but whenever their intellects were enlightened, and their sentiments roused, to appreciate the advantages of adopting, and disadvantages of neglecting, the improvement, it became easy.

The truth of these views may be still further illustrated by examples. A young gentleman of Glasgow, whom I knew, went out, as a merchant to North America. Business required him to sail from New York to St. Domingo. The weather was hot, and he, being very sick, found the confinement below deck, in bed, as he said, intolerable; that is, this confinement was, for the moment, more painful than the course which he adopted, of laying himself down at full length on the deck, in the open air. He was warned by his fellow passengers, and the officers of the ship, that he would inevitably induce fever by this proceeding: but he was utterly ignorant of the physical and organic laws; his intellect had been trained to regard only wealth and present pleasure as objects of real importance; it could perceive no necessary connexion between exposure to the mild and grateful sea breeze of a warm climate and fever, and he obstinately refused to quit his position. The consequence was, that he was rapidly taken ill, and lived just one day after arriving at St. Domingo. Knowledge of chemistry and physiology would have enabled him, in an instant, to understand that the sea air, in warm climates, holds a prodigious quantity of water in solution, and that damp and heat, operating together on the human organs, tend to derange their healthy action, and ultimately to destroy them entirely: and if his sentiments had been deeply imbued with a feeling of the indispensable duty of yielding obedience to the institutions of the Creator, he would have actually enjoyed, not only a *greater desire*, but a *greater power* of supporting the temporary inconvenience of the heated cabin, and might, by possibility, have escaped death.

Captain MURRAY, R. N. mentioned to Dr. A. COMBE, that, in his opinion, most of the bad effects of the climate of the West Indies might be avoided by care and attention to clothing; and so satisfied was he on this point, that he had petitioned to be sent there in preference to the North American station, and had no reason to regret the change. The measures which he adopted, and their effects, are detailed in the following interesting and instructive letter:

'*Assynt, April* 22, 1827.

' My Dear Sir,

' I should have written to you before this, had I not been anxious to refer to some memorandums, which I could not do before my return home from Coul. I attribute the great good health enjoyed by the crew of his Majesty's ship Valorous, when on the West India station, during the period I had the honour of commanding her, to the following causes. 1st, To the keeping the ship perfectly *dry* and *clean;* 2dly, To habituating the men to the wearing of flannel *next* the *skin;* 3dly, To the precaution I adopted, of giving each man a proportion of his allowance of cocoa *before* he left the ship in the *morning*, either for the purpose of watering, or any other duty he might be sent upon; and, 4thly, To the cheerfulness of the crew.

' The Valorous sailed from Plymouth on the 24th December, 1823, having just returned from the coast of Labrador and Newfoundland, where she had been stationed two years, the crew, including officers, amounting to 150 men. I had ordered the purser to draw two pairs of flannel drawers, and two shirts extra for each man, as soon as I knew that our destination was the West Indies; and, on our sailing, I issued two of each to every man and boy in the ship, making the officers of each division responsible for the men of their respective divisions wearing these flannels during the day and night; and, at the regular morning nine o'clock musters, I inspected the crew personally; for you can hardly conceive the difficulty I have had in *forcing* some of the men to use flannel at first; although I never yet knew one who did not, from choice, adhere to it, when once fairly adopted. The only precaution after this, was to *see* that, in bad weather, the watch, when relieved, did not turn in, in their wet clothes, which the young hands were apt to do, if not looked after; and their flannels were shifted every Sunday.

'Whenever fresh beef and vegetables could be procured at the contract price, they were always issued in preference to salt provision. Lime juice was issued whenever the men had been fourteen days on ship's provisions; and the crew took their meals on the main deck, except in very bad weather.

'The quarter and main decks were scrubbed with sand and water, and wet holy stones, every morning at daylight. The lower deck, cock-pit, and store-rooms were scrubbed every day after breakfast, with dry holy stones and hot sand, until quite *white*, the sand being carefully swept up, and thrown overboard. The pump-well was also swabbed out dry, and then scrubbed with holy stones and hot sand; and here, as well as in every part of the ship which was liable to damp, Brodiestoves were constantly used, until every appearance of humidity vanished. The lower deck and cock-pit were washed once every week in dry weather; but Brodiestoves were constantly kept burning in them, until they were quite dry again.

'The hammocks were piped up, and in the nettings, from 7 A. M. until dusk, when the men of each watch took down their hammocks alternately, by which means, only one half of the hammocks being down at a time, the tween decks were not so crowded, and the watch relieved was sure of turning into a dry bed on going below. The bedding was aired every week, once at least. The men were not permitted to go on shore in the heat of the sun, or where there was a probability of their getting *spirituous liquors;* but all hands were indulged with a run on shore, when out of reach of such temptation.

'I was employed on the Coast of Caraccas, the West India Islands, and Gulf of Mexico; and in course of service, I visited Trinidad, Margarita, Cocha, Cumana, Nueva Barcelona, Laguira, Porto Cabello, and Maracaibo, on the coast of Caraccas; all the West India Islands, from Tobago to Cuba, both inclusive; as also, Caracao and Aruba, and several of those places repeatedly; also to Vera Cruz and Tampico, in the Gulf of Mexico, which you will admit must have given a trial to the constitutions of my men, after two years amongst the icebergs of the Labrador, without an intervening summer between that icy coast and the coast of Caraccas; yet I arrived in England on June 24th, without having buried a single man or officer belonging to the ship, or indeed having a single man on the sick list; from which I am satisfied that a *dry* ship will always be a healthy one in any climate. When in command of the Recruit, of 18 guns, in the year 1809, I was sent to Vera Cruz, where I found the ———— 46, the ———— 42, the ————18, and ———— gun-brig; we were joined by the ———— 36, and the ———— 18. During the period we remained at anchor (from 8 to 10 weeks), the three frigates lost from 30 to 50 men each, the brigs 16 to 18, the ———— most of her crew, with two different commanders; yet the Recruit, although moored in the middle of the squadron, and constant intercourse held with the other ships, did not lose a man, and had none sick. Now, as some of these ships had been as long in the West Indies as the Recruit, we cannot attribute her singular healthy state to *seasoning*, nor can I to superior cleanliness, because even the breeches of the carronades, and all the pins, were polished bright in both ———— and ————, which was not the case with the Recruit. Perhaps her healthy state may be attributed to cheerfulness in the men; to my never allowing them to go on shore in the morning, on an empty stomach; to the use of dry sand and holy stone for the ship; to never working them in the sun; perhaps to accident. Were I asked my opinion, I would say that I firmly believe that cheerfulness contributes more to keep a ship's company healthy, than any precaution that can be adopted; and that, with this attainment, combined with the precautions I have mentioned, I should sail for the West Indies, with as little anxiety as I would for any other station. My Valorous fellows were as cheerful a set as I ever saw collected together.'

Suppose that two gontlemen were to ascend one of the Scottish mountains, in a hot summer day, and to arrive at the top, bathed in perspiration, and exhausted with fatigue. That one of them knew intimately the physical and organic laws, and that, all hot and wearied as he was, he should button up his coat closer about his body, wrap a handkerchief about his neck and continue walking, at a quick pace, round the summit, in the full blaze of the sun. That the other, ignorant of these laws, should eagerly run to the base of a projecting cliff; stretch himself at full length on the turf, under its refreshing shade; open his vest to the grateful breeze; and, in short, give himself up entirely to the present luxuries of coolness and repose;—the former, by warding off the rapid chill of the cool mountain air, would descend with health unimpaired; while the latter would carry with him, to a certainty, the seeds of rheumatism, consumption, or fever, from permitting perspiration to be instantaneously checked, and the surface of the body to be cooled with an injurious rapidity. I have put these cases hypothetically, because, although I have seen and experienced the benefits of the former method, I have not directly observed the opposite. No season, however, passes in the Highlands, in which some tragedy of the latter description does not occur; and, from the minutest information that I have been able to obtain, the causes have been such as are here described.

I shall conclude these examples by a case which is illustrative of the points under consideration, and which I have too good an opportunity of observing in all its stages.

An individual in whom it was my duty as well as pleasure, to be greatly interested, had resolved on carrying Mr. Owen's views into practical effect, and got an establishment set agoing on his principles, at Orbiston, in Lanarkshire. The labour and anxiety which he underwent at the commencement of the undertaking, gradually impaired an excellent constitution; and, without perceiving the change, he, by way of setting an example of industry, took to digging with the spade, and actually worked fourteen days at this occupation, although previously unaccustomed to labour. This produced hæmoptysis. Being unable now for bodily exertion, he gave up his whole time to directing and instructing the people, about 250 in number, and for two or three weeks *spoke the whole day*, the effusion from his lungs continuing. Nature rapidly sunk under this irrational treatment; and at last he came to Edinburgh for medical advice. When the structure and uses of his lungs were explained to him, and when it was pointed out that his treatment of them had been equally injudicious as if he had thrown lime or dust into his eyes, after inflammation, he was struck with the extent and consequences of his own ignorance, and exclaimed, How greatly he would have been benefited if one month of the five years which he had been forced to spend in a vain attempt at acquiring a mastery over the Latin tongue, had been dedicated to conveying to him information concerning the structure of his body, and the causes which preserve and impair its functions. He had departed too widely from the organic laws to admit of an easy return; he was seized with inflammation of the lungs, and with great difficulty got through that attack; but it impaired his constitution so grievously, that he died, after a lingering illness of eleven months. He acknowledged, however, even in his severest pain, that he suffered under a just law. The lungs, he saw, were of the first-rate importance to life, and their proper treatment was provided for by this tremendous punishment, inflicted for neglecting the conditions requisite to their health. Had he given them rest, and returned to obedience to the organic law, at the first intimation of departure from it, the door stood wide open and ready to receive him; but, in utter ignorance, he persevered for weeks in direct opposition to these conditions, till the fearful result ensued.

This last case affords a striking illustration of the independence of the different institutions of the Creator, and of the necessity of obeying *all* of them, as the only condition of safety and enjoyment. The individual here alluded to, was deeply engaged in a most benevolent and disinterested experiment for promoting the welfare of his fellow creatures; and superficial observers would say that this was just an example of the inscrutable decrees of Providence, which visited him with sickness, and ultimately with death, in the very midst of his most virtuous exertions. But the institutions of the Creator are wiser than the imaginations of such men. The first principle on which existence on earth, and all its advantages depend, is obedience to the physical and organic laws. The benevolent Owenite neglected these, in his zeal to obey the moral law; and, if it were possible to dispense with the one, by obeying the other, the whole theatre of man's existence would speedily become deranged, and involved in inexplicable disorder.

Having traced bodily sufferings, in the case of individuals, to neglect of, or opposition to, the organic laws, by their progenitors or by themselves, I next advert to another set of calamities, that may be called social miseries, and which obviously spring from the same causes; but of which latter fact complete evidence was not possessed until Phrenology was discovered. And, first, in regard to evils of a domestic nature;—One fertile source of unhappiness arises from persons uniting in marriage whose tempers, talents, and dispositions do not harmonize. If it be true that natural talents and dispositions are connected by the Creator with particular configurations of brain, then it is obviously one of His institutions that, in forming a compact for life, these should be attended to.* If we imagine an individual endowed with the splendid cerebral developement of Raphael, under a mere animal impulse, uniting himself for life with a female, possessing a brain like that of Mary Macinnes,† which by no possibility, could sympathise with his, this proceeding would be as direct an obstacle to happiness, as if a man were to surround himself with ice to remove sensations of cold. Until Phrenology was discovered, no natural index to mental qualities, that could be practically relied on, was possessed, and each individual was left to his own sagacity in directing his conduct; but the natural law never bended one iota to accommodate itself to that state of ignorance. The Creator having bestowed on mankind faculties fitted to discover Phrenology, having constituted them so that their greatest enjoyment should consist in activity, framed his institutions in such a way as to confer happiness when they were discovered, and observed, and to carry punishment when unknown and infringed, as an arrangement at once benevolent and wise for the race. If it be the fact, that natural talents and dispositions are indicated by cerebral developement; and if an individual, after this truth reaches his mind, shall form a connexion fitted to occasion him sorrow, it is obvious he must do so from one of two causes, either from contempt of the effects of developement of brain, and a secret belief that he may evade its consequences, which is just contempt of an organic law, and disbelief in its consequences; or, secondly, from the predominance of avarice, or some animal or other feeling precluding his yielding obedience to what he sees to

---

* See Appendix, Note 2.
† Casts of these heads are sold in the shops, and will be found in many Phrenological collections.

be an institution of the Creator. In either case, he must abide the consequences; and although these may be grievous, they cannot be complained of as unjust. In the play of the Gamester, Mrs. Beverly is represented as a most excellent wife, acting habitually under the guidance of the moral sentiments and intellect; but she is married to a being who, while he adores her, reduces her to beggary and misery. His sister utters an exclamation to this effect:— Why did just heaven unite such an angel to so heartless a thing! The parallel of this case occurs too often in real life; only it is not 'just Heaven' that makes such matches, but ignorant and thoughtless human beings, who imagine themselves absolved from all obligation to study and obey the natural laws of Heaven, as announced in the general arrangement of the universe. Phrenology will put it in the power of mankind to mitigate these evils, when they choose to adopt its dictates as a practical rule of conduct.

The justice and benevolence of rendering the individuals themselves unhappy who neglect this great institution of the Creator, become more striking when in the next place, we consider the effects, by the organic law, of such conduct on the children of these ill-assorted unions.

Physiologists, in general, are agreed, that a vigorous and healthy constitution of body in the parents, communicates existence, in the most perfect state, to the offspring,* and many observers of mankind, as well as medical authors, have remarked, also, the transmission, by hereditary descent, of mental talents and dispositions.

Dr. KING, in speaking of the fatality which attended the House of Stuart, says, 'If I were to ascribe their calamities to another cause (than an evil fate), or endeavour to account for them by any natural means, I should think they

---

* Very young hens lay small eggs; but a breeder of fowls will never set these to be hatched, because the animals produced would be feeble and imperfectly developed. They select the largest and freshest eggs, and endeavour to rear the healthiest stock possible.

were chiefly owing to a certain *obstinacy of temper*, which appears to have *been hereditary and inherent* in all the Stuarts, except Charles II.

It is well known that the caste of the Brahmins is the highest in point of intelligence as well as rank of all the castes in Hindostan; and it is mentioned by the missionaries as an ascertained fact, that *their* children are naturally more acute, intelligent, and docile, than the children of the inferior castes, age and other circumstances being equal.

Dr. Gregory, in treating of the temperaments in his *Conspectus Medicinæ Theoreticæ*, says, ' Hujusmodi varietates non corpori smodò, verùm et animi quoque, plerumque congenitæ, nonnunquam hæreditariæ, observantur. Hoc modo parentes sæpe in proles reviviscunt; certè parentibus liberi similes sunt, non vultum modò et corporis formam, sed animi indolem, et virtutes, et vitia. Imperiosa gens Claudia diu Romæ floruit, impigra, ferox, superba; eadem illachrymabilem Tiberium, tristissimum tyrennum, produxit; tandem in immanem Caligulam, et Claudium, et Agrippinam, ipsumque demum Neronem, post sexcentos annos, desitura.'*—Cap. i. sect. 16.

Phrenology reveals the principle on which these phenomena take place. Mental talents and dispositions are determined by the size and constitution of the brain. The brain is a portion of our organized system, and as such, is subject to the organic laws, by one of which its qualities are transmitted by hereditary descent. This law, however, faint or obscure it may appear in individual cases, becomes absolutely undeniable in nations. When we place the collection of Hindoo, Charib, Negro, New Holland, North American, and European skulls, possessed by the Phrenological Society, in juxtaposition, we perceive a na-

---

* Parents frequently live again in their offspring. It is quite certain that children resemble their parents, not only in countenance and the form of their body, bu. also in their mental dispositions, in their virtues and vices, &c.

tional form and combination of organs in each actually obtruding itself upon our notice, and corresponding with the mental characters of the respective tribes; the cerebral developement of one tribe is seen to differ as widely from that of another, as the European mind does from that of the New Hollander. Here, then, each Hindoo, Chinese, New Hollander, Negro, and Charib, obviously inherits from his parents a certain general type of head; and so does each European. If, then, the general forms and proportions are thus so palpably transmitted, can we doubt that the individual varieties follow the same rule, modified slightly by causes peculiar to the parents of the individual? The differences of national *character* are equally conspicuous as those of national *brains*, and it is surprising how permanently both endure. It is observed by an author in the *Edinburgh Review*, that 'the Vicentine district is, as every one knows, and has been for ages, an integral part of the Venetian dominions, professing the same religion, and governed by the same laws, as the other continental provinces of Venice; yet the English character is not more different from the French, than that of the Vicentine from the Paduan; while the contrast between the Vicentine and his other neighbour, the Veronese, is hardly less remarkable.'—No. lxxxiv. p. 459.

If, then, form, size, and constitution of brain, are transmitted from parents to children, if these determine natural mental talents and dispositions, which in their turn exercise the greatest influence over the happiness of individuals through the whole of life, it becomes extremely important to discover according to what laws this transmission takes place. Three principles present themselves to our consideration, at the first aspect of the question. Either in the first place, the constitution and qualities of brain, which the parents themselves inherit at birth, are transmitted absolutely, so that the children, sex following sex, are exact copies, without variation or modification, of the one parent or the other; or, secondly, the natural and inherent qualities of the father and mother combine, and are transmitted in a modified form to the offspring; or, thirdly, the qualities of the children are determined jointly by the constitution of the stock, and by the faculties which predominate in power and activity in the parents, at the particular time when the organic existence of each child commences.

Experience shows that the *first* cannot be the law; for, as often mentioned, a real law of nature admits of no exceptions, and it is well established, that the minds of children are *not exact* copies, without variation or modification, of those of the parents, sex following sex. Neither can the second be the law, because it is equally certain that the minds of children, although *sometimes, are not always,* in talents and disposition, perfect modifications of those of the father and mother. If this law prevailed, no child would be a copy of the father, none a copy of the mother, nor of any collateral relation, but each would be invariably a compound of the two parents, and all the children would be exactly alike, sex only excepted. . Experience shows, that this cannot be the law. What, then, does experience say to the *third* idea, that the mental character of each child is determined by the particular qualities of the stock, combined with those which predominate in the parents, when its existence commenced.

I have already adverted to the influence of the stock, and shall now illustrate that of the condition of the parents, when existence is communicated.

A strong illustration, in the case of the lower animals, appeared in the Edinburgh Review, No. lxxxiv. p. 457.

'Every one conversant with beasts,' says the reviewer, 'knows, that not only their natural, but that many of their acquired qualities, are transmitted by the parents to their offspring. Perhaps the most curious example of the latter fact may be found in the pointer.

'This animal is endowed with the natural instinct of winding game, and stealing upon his prey, which he surprises, having first made a short pause, in order to launch himself upon it with more security of success. This sort of *semicolon* in his proceedings, man converts into a *full stop*, and teaches him to be as much pleased at seeing the bird or beast drop by the shooter's gun, as at taking it himself. The staunchest dog of this kind, and of the original pointer, is of Spanish origin, and our own is derived from this race, crossed with that of the foxhound, or other breed of dog, for the sake of improving his speed. This mixed and factitious race, of course, naturally partakes less of the true pointer character; that is to say, is less disposed to stop, or at least he makes a shorter stop at game. The *factitious pointer is, however, disciplined, in this country, into staunchness; and, what is most singular,* THIS QUALITY IS, IN A GREAT DEGREE, INHERITED BY HIS PUPPY, who may be seen earnestly standing at swallows or pigeons in a farm yard. For intuition, though it leads the offspring to exercise his parent's faculties, does not instruct him how to direct them. The preference of his master afterwards guides him in his selection, and teaches him what game is better worth pursuit. On the other hand, the pointer of pure Spanish race, unless he happen to be well broke himself, which in the south of Europe seldom happens, produces a race which are all but unteachable, according to our notions of a pointer's business. They will make a stop at their game, as natural instinct prompts them, but seem incapable of being drilled into the habits of the animal, which education has formed in this country, and has rendered, as I have said, in some degree, capable of transmitting his acquirements to his descendants.

'Acquired habits are hereditary in other animals besides dogs. English sheep, probably from the greater richness of our pastures, feed very much together; while Scotch sheep are obliged to extend and scatter themselves over their hills for the better discovery of food. Yet the English sheep, on being transferred to Scotland, *keep their old habit of feeding in a mass,* though so little adapted to their new country; so do their descendants; and the English sheep is not thoroughly naturalized into the necessities of his place *till the third generation.* The same thing may be observed as to the nature of his food, that is observed in his mode of seeking it. When turnips were introduced from England into Scotland, *it was only the third generation* which heartily adopted this diet, the first having been starved into an acquiescence in it.'

In these instances, long continued impressions on the parents appear to have at last effected change of disposition in the offspring.

'We have seen,' says an author whom I have already quoted, 'how wonderfully the *bee* works—according to rules discovered by man thousands of years after the insect had followed them with perfect accuracy. The same little animal seems to be acquainted with principles of which we are still ignorant. We can, by crossing, vary the forms of cattle with astonishing nicety; but we have no means of altering the nature of an animal, once born, by means of treatment and feeding. This power, however, is undeniably possessed by the bees. When the queen-bee is lost, by death or otherwise, they chocse a grub from among those who are born for workers; they make three cells into one, and, placing the grub there, they build a tube round it; they afterwards build another cell, of a pyramidal form, into which the grub grows: they feed it with peculiar food, and tend it with extreme care. It becomes, when transformed from the worm to the fly, not a worker, but a queen-bee.'—*Objects, Advantages, and Pleasures of Science,* p. 33. It is difficult to conceive that man will ever possess such a power as this last.

Man, however, as an organized being, is subject to laws similar to those which govern the organization of the lower animals. Dr. Pritchard, in his researches into the Physical History of Mankind, has brought forward a variety of interesting facts and opinions on this subject of transmission of hereditary qualities in the human race. He says, 'Children resemble, in feature and constitution, both parents, but, I think more generally the father. In the breeding of horses and oxen, great importance is attached, by experienced propagators, to the male. In sheep it is commonly observed that black rams beget black lambs. In the human species, also, the complexion chiefly follows that of the father; and I believe it to be a general fact, that the offspring of a *black father* and white mother is *much darker* than the progeny of a *white father* and a black mother.'—Vol. ii. p. 551. These facts appear to me to be referable to both causes. The stock must have had some influence, but the mother, in all these cases, is not impressed by her own colour, because she does not look on herself; while the *father's* complexion must strikingly attract her attention, and may, in this way, give the darker tinge to the offspring.*

Dr. Pritchard states the result of his investigations to be, First, That the organization of the offspring is always modelled according to the type of the *original structure* of the parent; and, Secondly, 'That changes, produced by external causes in the appearance or constitution of the individual are temporary; and, in general, acquired characters are transient; they terminate with the individual, and have no influence on the progeny.'—Vol. ii. p. 536. He supports the first of these propositions by a variety of facts occurring ' in the porcupine family,' ' in the hereditary nature of complexion,' and, ' in the growth of supernumerary fingers or toes, and corresponding deficiencies.' ' Maupertuis has mentioned this phenomenon; he assures us, that there were two families in Germany, who have been

---

* Black hens lay dark-coloured eggs.

distinguished for several generations by six fingers on each hand, and the same number of toes on each foot,' &c. He admits, at the same time, that the *second* proposition is of more difficult proof, and that an opinion contrary to it 'has been maintained by some writers, and a variety of singular facts have been related in support of it.' But many of these relations, as he justly observes, are obviously fables.

In regard to the foregoing propositions, I would observe, that a manifest distinction exists between transmission of monstrosities, or mutilations, which constitute additions to, or abstractions from, the natural lineaments of the body, and transmission of a mere tendency in particular organs to a greater or less developement of their natural functions. This last appears to me to be influenced by the state of the parents, at the time when existence is communicated to the offspring. On this point Dr. PRITCHARD says, 'The opinion which formerly prevailed, and which has been entertained by some modern writers, among whom is Dr. DARWIN, that at the period when organization commences in the ovum, that is, at or soon after the time of conception, the structure of the fœtus is capable of undergoing modification from impressions on the mind or senses of the parent, does not appear altogether so improbable. It is contradicted, at least, by no fact in physiology. It is an opinion of very ancient prevalence, and may be traced to so remote a period, that its rise cannot be attributed to the speculations of philosophers, and it is difficult to account for the origin of such a persuasion, unless we ascribe it to facts which happened to be observed.' p. 556.

A striking and undeniable proof of the effect on the character and dispositions of children, produced by the form of brain transmitted to them by hereditary descent, is to be found in the progeny of marriages between Europeans, whose brains possess a favourable developement of the moral and intellectual organs, and Hindoos, and native

Americans, whose brains are inferior. All authors agree, and report the circumstance as singularly striking, that the children of such unions are decidedly superior in mental qualities to the native, while they are still inferior to the European parent. Captain FRANKLIN says, that the half-breed American Indians 'are upon the whole a good looking people; and where the experiments have been made, have shown much expertness in learning, and willingness to be taught; they have, however, been sadly neglected, p. 36. He adds, 'It has been remarked, I do not know with what truth, that half breeds show more personal courage than the pure breeds.' Captain BASIL HALL, and other writers on South America, mention that the offspring of native American and Spanish parents, constitute the most active, vigorous, and powerful portion of the inhabitants of these countries; and many of them rose to high commands during the revolutionary war. So much is this the case in Hindostan, that several writers have already pointed to the mixed race there, as obviously destined to become the future sovereigns of India. These individuals inherit from the native parent a certain adaptation to the climate, and from the European parent a higher developement of brain, the two combined constituting their superiority.

Another example of the same law occurs in Persia. In that country, it is said that the custom has existed for ages among the nobles, of purchasing beautiful female Circassian captives, and forming alliances with them as wives. It is ascertained that the Circassian form of brain stands comparatively high in the developement of the moral and intellectual organs.* And it is mentioned by some travellers, that the race of nobles in Persia is the most gifted in

---

* In Mr. W. ALLAN's picture of the Circassian Captives, the form of the head is said to be a copy from nature, taken by that artist, when he visited the country. It is engraved by Mr. JAMES STEWART with great beauty and fidelity, and may be consulted as an example of the superiority of Circassian developement of the brain.

natural qualities, bodily and mental, of any class of that people; a fact diametrically opposite to that which takes place in Spain, and other European countries, where the nobles intermarry constantly with each other, and set the organic laws altogether at defiance.

The degeneracy and even idiocy of some of the noble and royal families of Spain and Portugal, from marrying nieces, and other near relations, is well known; and defective brains, in all these cases, are observed.

The father of Napoleon Bonaparte, says Sir Walter Scott, ' is stated to have possessed a very handsome person, a talent for eloquence, and a vivacity of intellect, which he transmitted to his son.' ' It was in the middle of civil discord, fights, and skirmishes, that Charles Bonaparte married Lætitia Ramolini, one of the most beautiful young women of the island, and possessed of a great deal of firmness of character. She partook of the dangers of her husband during the years of civil war, and is said to have accompanied him on horseback on some military expeditions, or perhaps hasty flights, shortly before her being delivered of the future Emperor.'—*Life of* Napoleon Bonaparte, vol. iii. p. 6.

The murder of David Rizzio was perpetrated by armed nobles, with many circumstances of violence and terror, in the presence of Mary, Queen of Scotland, shortly before the birth of her son, afterwards James the First of England. The constitutional liability of this monarch to emotions of fear, is recorded as a characteristic of his mind; and it has even been mentioned that he started involuntarily at the sight of a drawn sword. Queen Mary was not deficient in courage, and the Stuarts, both before and after James the First, were distinguished for this quality; so that he was a marked exception to the dispositions of his family. Napoleon and James form striking contrasts; and it may be remarked that the mind of Napoleon's mother appears to have risen to the danger to which she was exposed, and braved it; while the circumstances in which Queen Mary was placed, were calculated to inspire her with fear alone.

Further evidence of the same law may still be mentioned. Esquirol, the celebrated French medical writer, in adverting to the causes of madness, mentions that many children whose existence dated from periods when the horrors of the French Revolution were at their height, turned out subsequently to be weak, nervous, and irritable in mind, extremely susceptible of impressions, and liable, by the least extraordinary excitement, to be thrown into absolute insanity. Again, in a case which fell under my observation, the father of a family was sick, had a partial recovery, but relapsed, declined, and in two months died. Seven months after his death, a son was born, of the full age; and the origin of whose existence was referable to the period of the partial recovery. At that time, and during the subsequent two months, the faculties of the mother were in the highest state of excitement, in ministering to her husband, to whom she was greatly attached; and, after his death, the same excitement continued to operate, for she was then loaded with the charge of a numerous family, but not depressed; for her circumstances were comfortable. The child is now more than ten years old; and, while his constitution is the most delicate, his developement of the mental organs, and the natural activity of these, is decidedly the greatest of the family. Another illustration of the same law is found in the fact, that, when two parties marry very young, the eldest of their children generally inherits a less favourable developement of the moral and intellectual organs, than those produced in more mature age,—which is in exact correspondence with the doctrine, that the animal faculties in men, in general, are most vigorous in early life, and will then be most readily transmitted to offspring. Indeed, it appears difficult to account for the wide varieties in the form of the brain in children of the same family, unless on the principle, that the organs which predominate in activity and vigour in the parents, at the time when existence is communicated, determine the tendency of corresponding organs to develope themselves largely in the children. If this is really the law of nature, as there is great reason for believing, then parents, in whom combativeness and destructiveness are in habitual activity, will transmit these organs, in a state of high developement and excitement, to their children; and those in whom the moral and intellectual organs exist in supreme vigour, will transmit these in greatest perfection.

This view is in harmony with the fact that children generally, although not universally, resemble the parents in their mental qualities; because the largest organs being naturally the most active, the general and habitual state of the parents will be strongly marked by those which predominate in size in their own brain; and on the principle of predominance in activity and energy causing the transmission of similar qualities to the offspring, the children will, in this way, very generally resemble the parents. But they will not always do so; because, even MARY MACINNES, in whom the moral and intellectual organs were extremely deficient, might have been exposed to external influences, which, for the time being, might have excited them to unwonted vivacity; and, according to the rule, as now explained, a child, dating its existence from that period, might have inherited a higher organization of brain than her own. Or, a person with a very excellent moral developement, might, by some particular occurrence, have his animal propensities roused to unwonted vigour, and his moral sentiments thrown, for the time, into the shade; and any offspring connected with that condition, would prove inferior to himself in the developement of the moral organs, and greatly surpass him in the size of those of the propensities.

I do not present these views as ascertained phrenological science, but as inferences strongly supported by facts, and consistent with known phenomena. If we suppose them to be true, they will greatly strengthen the motives for preserving the *habitual* supremacy of the moral sentiments and intellect, when, by doing so, improved moral and intellectual capacities may be conferred on offspring. If it be true that this lower world, so far as man is concerned, is framed to harmonize with the supremacy of the higher faculties of the mind, what a noble prospect would this law open up of the possibility of man ultimately becoming capable of placing himself more fully in accordance with the Divine institutions, than he has hitherto been able to accomplish; and, in consequence, of reaping numberless enjoyments that appear destined for him by his Creator, and avoiding thousands of miseries that now render his life a series of calamities. The views here expounded also harmonize with the second principle of this Essay, namely, That, as activity in the faculties is the fountain of enjoyment, the whole constitution of nature is designedly framed to call on them for ceaseless exertion. What scope for observation, reflection, the exercise of moral sentiments, and regulating of animal impulse, does not this picture of nature present!

I cordially agree, however, with Dr. Pritchard, that this subject is still involved in very great obscurity. 'We know not,' says he, ' by what means any of the facts we remark are effected; and the utmost we can hope to attain, is, by tracing the connexions of circumstances, to learn from what combinations of them we may expect to witness particular results.'—Vol. ii. p. 542. But much of the darkness may be traced to the past ignorance of mankind concerning the functions of the brain. If we consider that it has all along been the most important organ of our system; that, from its office, mental impressions must almost necesarrily have exercised a powerful influence over the developement of its parts, and that the relative size of these determines the predominance of particular talents and dispositions; but, nevertheless, that all past observations have been conducted without the knowledge of these principles; it will not appear marvellous that merely confusion and contradiction have existed in the results drawn. At the present moment, accordingly, almost all that phrenologists can pretend to accomplish, is, to point out the mighty void; to offer an exposition of its causes; and to state such inferences as their own very limited observations have hitherto enabled them to deduce. Far from pretending to be in possession of certain and complete knowledge on this subject, I am inclined to think, that, although every conjecture now hazarded were true, several centuries of observation will probably be required to render the principles completely practical. At present we have almost no information concerning the effects, on the children, of different temperaments, of different combinations in the cerebral organs, of differences of age, &c., in the parents.

It is astonishing, however, to what extent mere pecuniary interests excite men to investigate and observe the Natural Laws, and how small an influence moral and rational considerations exert in leading them to do so. Before a common insurance company will undertake the risk of paying £100, on the death of an individual, they require the following questions to be answered by credible and intelligent witnesses:

'1. How long have you known Mr. A. B.?
'2. Has he had the gout?
'3. Has he had a spitting of blood, asthma, consumption, or other pulmonary complaint?
'4. Do you consider him at all predisposed to any of these complaints?
'5. Has he been afflicted with fits, or mental derangement?
'6. Do you think his constitution perfectly good, in the common acceptation of the term?

' 7. Are his habits in every respect strictly regular and temperate?

' 8. Is he at present in good health?

' 9. Is there anything in his form, habits of living, or business, which you are of opinion may shorten his life?

' 10. What complaints are his family most subject to?

' 11. Are you aware of any reason why an insurance might not with safety be effected on his life?'

A man and woman about to marry, have in the general case, the health and happiness of five or more human beings depending on their attention to consideration, essentially the same as the foregoing, and yet how much less scrupulous are they than the mere speculators in money?

There is no moral difficulty in admitting and admiring the wisdom and benevolence of the institution, by which good qualities are transmitted from parents to children; but it is frequently held as unjust to the latter, that they should inherit parental deficiencies, and so be made to suffer for sins which they did not commit. In solving this difficulty, I must again refer to the supremacy of the moral sentiments, as the theory of the constitution of the world. The animal propensities are all selfish, and regard only the immediate and apparent interest of the individual; while the higher sentiments delight in that which communicates the greatest quantity of enjoyment to the greatest number. Now, let us suppose the law of hereditary descent to be abrogated altogether, that is to say, that each individual of the race at birth were endowed with fixed natural qualities, without the slightest reference to what his parents had been, or done;—this form of constitution would obviously cut off every possibility of improvement *in the race.* Every phrenologist knows, that the New Hollanders, Charibs, and other savage tribes, are distinguished by great deficiencies in the moral and intellectual organs.* If, however it

---

* This fact is demonstrated by specimens in most Phrenological Collections.

be true, that considerable developement of intellectual organs is indispensable to the comprehension of science, and the practice of virtue, it would, on the present supposition, be impossible to raise the New Hollanders, as a people, one step higher in capacity for intelligence and virtue than they now are. We might cultivate each generation up to the limit of its powers, but there the improvement, and a low one it would be, would stop; for the next generation, being produced with brains equally deficient in the moral and intellectual regions, no principle of increasing amelioration would exist. The same remarks are applicable to every tribe of mankind. If we assume modern Europeans as the standard, then, if the law of hereditary descent were abrogated, every deficiency that at this moment is attributable to imperfect or disproportionate developement of brain, would be irremediable, and continue as long as the race existed. Each generation might be cultivated till the summit level of its capacities was attained, but there each succeeding generation would remain. When we contrast with this prospect the very opposite effects flowing from the law of hereditary transmission of qualities in an increasing ratio, the whole advantages are at once perceived to be on the side of the latter constitution. According to this rule, the children of the individuals who have obeyed the organic, the moral, and the intellectual laws, would start from the highest level of their parents, not only in acquired knowledge, but in consequence of that very obedience, they would inherit an enlarged developement of the moral and intellectual organs, and thereby enjoy an increasing capability of discovering and obeying the Creator's institutions. This improvement, will, no doubt, have its limits; but it may probably extend to that point at which man will be capable of placing himself in harmony with the natural laws. The effort necessary to *maintain* himself there, will still provide for the activity of his faculties.

2dly. We may suppose the law of hereditary descent to be limited to the transmission of good, and abrogated as to the transmission of bad qualities; and it may be thought that this arrangement would be more benevolent and just. There are objections to this view, however, which do not occur at once to the mind. We see as matter of fact, that a vicious and debased parent is actually defective in the moral and intellectual organs. Now, if his children should take up exactly the same developement as himself, this would be transmission of imperfections, which is the very point objected to; or, if he were to take up a developement fixed by nature, and not at all referable to that of the parent; this would render the whole race stationary in their first condition, without the possibility of improvement in their capacities, which also we have seen would be an evil greatly to be deprecated.

3dly. The bad developement might be supposed to transmit, by hereditary descent, a good developement; but this would set at naught the supremacy of justice and benevolence; it would render the consequences of contempt for, and violation of the divine laws, and of obedience to them, in this particular, precisely alike. The debauchee, the cheat, the murderer, and the robber, would, according to this view, be able to look upon the prospects of their prosperity, with the same confidence in their welfare and happiness, as the pious and intelligent Christian, who had sought to know God and to obey his institutions during his whole life. Certainly no individual, in whom the higher sentiments prevail, will for a moment regard this imagined change as any improvement on the Creator's arrangements. What a host of motives to moral and religious conduct would at once be withdrawn, were such a spectacle of divine government exhibited to the mind. In proportion as the brain is improved, the aptitude of man for discovering and obeying the natural laws will be increased. For example, it appears to me that the native American savages and native New Hollanders, cannot, with their present brains, adopt European civilization. The reader will find in the Phrenological Collections specimens of their skulls, and, on comparing them with those of Europeans, he will observe that, in the former, the organs of reflecting intellect, Ideality, Conscientiousness, and Benevolence, are greatly inferior in size to the same organs in the latter. If, by obeying the organic laws, the moral and intellectual organs of these savages could be considerably enlarged, they would *desire* civilization, and would adopt it when offered. If this view be well founded, all means used for their cultivation, which are not calculated at the same time to improve their cerebral organization, will be limited in their effects by the narrow capacities attending their present developement. In youth, all the organs of the body are more susceptible of modification than in advanced age; and hence the effects of education on the young may arise from the greater susceptibility of the brain to impressions at that period than later.

4thly. It may be supposed that human happiness would have been more completely secured, by endowing all individuals at birth with that degree of developement of the moral and intellectual organs, which would have best fitted them for discovering and obeying the Creator's institutions, and by preventing all aberrations from this standard; just as the lower animals appear to have received instincts and capacities, adjusted with the most perfect wisdom to their conditions. Two remarks occur on this supposition. First; We are not competent at present to judge correctly how far the developement actually bestowed on the human race, is, or is not, wisely adapted to their circumstances; for there may, by possibility, be departments in the great system of human society, exactly suited to all existing forms of brain, not imperfect through disease, if our knowledge were sufficient to discover them. The want of a natural index to the mental dispositions and capacities of individuals, and of a philosophical theory of the constitution of society, has hitherto precluded the possibility of arriving at sound conclusions on this question. It appears to me probable, that while there may be great room for improvement in the talents and dispositions of vast numbers of individuals, the imperfections of the race in general may not be so great, as we, in our present state of ignorance of the aptitudes of particular persons for particular situations, are prone to infer. But, secondly, on the principle that activity in the faculties is the fountain of enjoyment, it may be considered whether additional motives to the exercise of the moral and intellectual powers, and, consequently, greater happiness, are not conferred by leaving men, within certain limits, to regulate the talents and tendencies of their descendants, than by endowing each individual with the best qualities, independently of the conduct of his parents.

On the whole, therefore, there seems reason for concluding, that the actual institution, by which both good and bad qualtities * are transmitted is, fraught with higher advantages to the race, than the abrogation of the law of transmission altogether; or than the supposed change of it, by which bad men would transmit good qualities to their children. The actual law, when viewed by the moral sentiments and intellect, both in its principles and consequences, appears beneficial and expedient. When an individual sufferer, therefore, complains of its operation, he regards it through the animal faculties alone; his self-love is annoy-

---

* In using the popular expressions ' good qualities' and ' bad qualities,' I do not mean to insinuate, that any of the tendencies bestowed on man are essentially bad in themselves. Destructiveness and Acquisitiveness, for example, are, when properly directed, unquestionably good; but they become the sources of evil, when their organs are too large, in proportion to those of the moral sentiments and intellect. By bad qualities, therefore, I always mean either disease, or unfavourable proportions among the different organs.

ed, and he carries his thoughts no further. He never stretches his mind forward to the consequences to mankind at large, if the law which grieves him were reversed. The animal faculties regard nothing beyond their own immediate and apparent interest, and they do not even discern it correctly; for no arrangement that is beneficial for the race can be injurious to individuals, if its operations in regard to them were distinctly traced.

The abrogation of the rule, therefore, under which they complain, would, we may be certain, bring ten thousand times greater evils, even upon themselves, than its continuance.

On the other hand, an individual sufferer under an hereditary pain, in whom the moral and intellectual faculties predominate, who should see the principle and consequences of the institution of hereditary descent, as now explained, would not murmur at them as unjust; he would bow with submission to an institution, which he perceived to be fraught with blessings to the race, when it was known and observed, and the very practice of this reverential acquiescence would be so delightful, that it would diminish, in a great degree, the severity of the evil. Besides, he would see the door of mercy standing widely open, and inviting his return; he would perceive that every step which he made in his own person towards exact obedience to the Creator's institutions, would remove by so much the organic penalty transmitted through his parents' transgressions, and that his posterity would reap the full benefits of his more dutiful observance.

It may be objected to the law of hereditary transmission of organic qualities, that the children of a blind and lame father have sound eyes and limbs: But, in the 1st place, these defects are generally the result of accident or disease, occurring either during pregnancy, or posterior to birth, and seldom or never the operation of nature; and, consequently, the original physical principles remaining entire in the constitution, the bodily imperfections are not transmitted to the progeny. 2dly. Where the defects are congenite or constitutional, it frequently happens that they are transmitted through successive generations. This is exemplified in deafness, in blindness, and even in the possession of supernumerary fingers or toes. The reason why such peculiarities are not transmitted to all the progeny, appears to be simply that, in general, only one parent is defective. If the father, for instance, be blind or deaf, the mother is generally free from that imperfection, and her influence naturally extends to, and modifies the result in, the progeny.

If the law of hereditary transmission of mental qualities be, as now explained, dependent on the organs in highest excitement in the parents, it will account for the varieties, along with the general resemblance, that occur in children of the same marriage. It will account also for the circumstance of genius being sometimes transmitted and sometimes not. Unless *both* parents possess the developements and temperament of genius, the law would not certainly transmit these qualities to the children; and even although both did possess these endowments, they would be transmitted only on condition of the parents obeying the organic laws, one of which forbids that excessive exertion of the mental and corporeal functions, which exhausts and debilitates the system; an error almost universally committed by persons endowed with high original talent, under the present condition of ignorance of the natural laws, and erroneous fashions and institutions of society. The supposed law would be disproved by cases of weak, imbecile, and vicious children, being born to parents whose own constitution and habits had been in the highest accordance with the organic, moral, and intellectual laws; but no such cases have hitherto come under my observation.

Further; after birth, it is quite certain that the organs most active in the parents have a decided tendency to cause and increase in the size of corresponding organs in the children, by habitually exciting and exercising them, which favours their growth. According to this law, habitual severity, chiding, and imperious conduct, proceeding from over-active Self-esteem and Destructiveness in the parents, rouse these faculties in the children, produce hatred and resistance, and increase the activity of the same organs, while those of the moral sentiments and intellect are left in a state of apathy.

Rules, however, are best taught by examples; and I shall, therefore, proceed to mention some facts that have fallen under my own notice, or been communicated to me from authentic sources, illustrative of the practical consequences of infringing the law of hereditary descent.

A man, aged about fifty, possessed a brain, in which the animal, moral, and knowing intellectual organs were all strong, but the reflecting weak. He was pious, but destitute of education; he married an unhealthy young woman, deficient in moral developement, but of considereble force of character; and several children were born. The father and mother were far from being happy; and, when the children attained to eighteen or twenty years of age, they were adepts in every species of immorality and profligacy; they picked their father's pockets, stole his goods, and got them sold back to him, by accomplices, for money, which was spent in betting and cock-fighting, drinking, and low debauchery. The father was heavily grieved; but knowing only two resources, he beat the children severely as long as he was able, and prayed for them; his own words were, that 'if, *after that*, it pleased the Lord to make vessels of wrath of them, the Lord's will must just be done.' I mention this last observation, not in jest, but in great seriousness. It was impossible not to pity the unhappy father; yet, who that sees the institutions of the Creator to be in themselves wise, but in this instance to have been directly violated, will not acknowledge that the bitter pangs of the poor old man were the consequences of his own ignorance; and that it was an erroneous view of the divine administration, which led him to overlook his own mistakes, and to attribute to the Almighty the purpose of making vessels of wrath of his children, as the only explanation which he could give of their wicked dispositions. Who that sees the cause of his misery must not lament that his piety should not have been enlightened by philosophy, and directed to obedience, in the first instance, to the organic institutions of the Creator, as one of the prescribed conditions, without observance of which he had no title to expect a blessing upon his offspring.

In another instance, a man, in whom the animal organs, particularly those of Combativeness and Destructiveness, were very large, but with a pretty fair moral and intellectual developement, married, against her inclination, a young woman, fashionably and showily educated, but with a very decided deficiency in Conscientiousness. They soon became unhappy, and even blows were said to have passed between them, although they belonged to the middle rank of life. The mother, in this case, employed the children to deceive and plunder the father, and, latterly, spent the produce in drink. The sons inherited the deficient morality of the mother, and the ill temper of the father. The family fireside became a theatre of war, and before the sons attained majority, the father was glad to get them removed from his house, as the only means by which he could feel even his life in safety from their violence; for they had by that time retaliated the blows with which he had visited them in their younger years; and he stated that he actually considered his life to be in danger from his own offspring.

In another family, the mother possesses an excellent developement of the moral and intellectual organs, while, in the father, the animal organs predominate in great excess. She has been the unhappy victim of ceaseless misfortune, originating from the misconduct of her husband. Some of the children have inherited the father's brain, and some the mother's; and of the sons whose heads resemble the father's, several have died through mere debauchery and profligacy under thirty years of age; whereas, those who resemble the mother are alive and little contaminated, even amidst all the disadvantages of evil example.

On the other hand, I am not acquainted with a single instance in which the moral and intellectual organs predominated in size, in both father and mother, and whose external circumstances also permitted their general activity, in which the *whole* children did not partake of a moral and intellectual character, differing slightly in degrees of excellence one from another, but all presenting the decided predominance of the human over the animal faculties.

There are well-known examples of the children of religious and moral fathers exhibiting dispositions of a very inferior description; but in all of these instances that I have been able to observe, there has been a large developement of the animal organs in the one parent, which was just controlled, but not much more, by the moral and intellectual powers: and in the other parent, the *moral* organs did not appear to be in large proportion. The unfortunate child inherited the large animal developement of the one, with the defective moral developement of the other; and, in this way, was inferior to both. The way to satisfy one's self on this point, is to examine the heads of the parents. In all such cases, a large base of the brain, which is the region of the animal propensities, will very probably be found in one or other of them.

Another organic law of the animal kingdom deserves attention; viz. that by which marriages betwixt blood relations tend decidedly to the deterioration of the physical and mental qualities of the offspring. In Spain kings marry their nieces, and in this country, first and second cousins marry without scruple; although every philosophical physiologist will declare that this is in direct opposition to the institutions of nature. This law holds also in the vegetable kingdom. 'A provision, of a very simple kind, is, in some cases, made to prevent the male and female blossoms of the same plant from breeding together, this being found to hurt the breed of vegetables, just as breeding in and in does the breed of animals. It is contrived, that the dust shall be shed by the male blossom before the female is ready to be affected by it, so that the impregnation must be performed by the dust of some other plant, and in this way the breed be crossed.'—*Objects, &c. of Science,* p. 33.

On the same principle, it is found highly advantageous in agriculture not to sow grain of the same stock in constant succession on the same soil. In individual instances, if the soil and plants are both possessed of great vigour and the highest qualities, the same kind of grain may be reaped in succession twice or thrice, with less perceptible deterioration than where these elements of reproduction are feeble and imperfect; and the same thing appears in the animal kingdom. If the first individuals connected in near relationship, who unite in marriage, are uncommonly robust, and possess very favourably developed brains, their offspring may not be so *much* deteriorated below the common standard of the country as to attract particular attention, and the law of nature is, in this instance, supposed not to hold; but it does hold, for to a law of nature there never is an exception. The offspring are uniformly inferior to what they *would have been,* if the parents had united with strangers in blood of *equal vigour and cerebral developement.* Whenever there is any remarkable deficiency in parents who are related in blood, these appear in the most marked and aggravated forms in the offspring. The fact is so well known, and so easily ascertained, that I forbear to enlarge upon it. So much for miseries arising from neglect of the organic laws in forming the *domestic compact.*

I proceed to advert to those evils which arise from overlooking the operation of the same laws in ordinary relations of society.

How many little annoyances arise from the misconduct of servants and dependents in various departments of life; how many losses, and sometimes ruin, arise from dishonesty and knavery in confidential clerks, partners, and agents. A mercantile house of great reputation, in London, was ruined and became bankrupt, by a clerk having embezzled a prodigious extent of funds, and absconded to America; another company in Edinburgh, was talked of about a year ago, which had sustained a great loss by a similar piece of dishonesty; a company in Paisley was ruined by one of the partners having collected the funds, and eloped with them to the United States; and lately, several bankers, and other persons, suffered severely in Edinburgh, by the conduct of an individual, some time connected with the public press. If it be true, then, that the mental qualities and dispositions of individuals are indicated and influenced by the developement of their brains, and that their actual conduct is the result of this developement, operated upon by their external circumstances, including in this latter every moral and intellectual influence coming from without, is it not obvious, that one and all of the evils here enumerated flowed from infringement of the natural institutions, that is to say, from having placed human beings decidedly deficient in moral or intellectual qualities in situations where these were required in a higher degree than they possessed them?

If any man were to go to sea in a paper boat, which the very fluidity of the element would dissolve, no one would be surprised at his being drowned: and, in like manner, if the Creator has constituted the brain so as to exert a great influence on the mental dispositions, and if, nevertheless, men are pleased to treat this fact with neglect and contempt, and to place individuals, naturally deficient in the moral organs, in situations where a great degree of these sentiments is required, they have no cause to be surprised if they suffer the penalties of their own misconduct, in being plundered and defrauded.

Although I can state, from experience, that it is possible, by the aid of Phrenology, to select individuals whose moral and intellectual qualities may be relied on, yet, the extremely limited extent of our practical knowledge in this respect fails to be confessed. To be able to judge accurately what combination of natural talents and dispositions in an individual will best fit him for any given employment, we require to have seen a variety of combinations tried in that particular department, and to have noted their effects. It is impossible, at least for me, to anticipate with unerring certainty, what these effects will be : but I have ever found nature constant ; and after once discovering, by experience, an assortment of qualities suited to a particular duty, I have found no subsequent exception to the rule. Cases in which the predominance of particular regions of the brain, as the moral and intellectual, is very decided, present fewest difficulties ; although, even in them, the very deficiency of animal organs may sometimes incapacitate an individual for important stations ; but where the three classes of organs, the animal, moral, and intellectual, are nearly *in æquilibrio*, the most opposite results may ensue by external circumstances exciting the one or the other to decided predominance in activity.

Having now adverted to calamities by external violence, —to bad health,—unhappiness in the domestic circle, arising from ill-advised unions, and viciously disposed children, —to the evils of placing individuals, as servants, clerks, partners, public instructers, &c., in situations to which they are not suited, by their natural qualities, and traced all of them to infringements or neglect of the physical or organic laws, I proceed to advert to the last, and what is reckoned the greatest of all calamities, DEATH, and which itself is obviously a part of the organic law. Baron Cuvier, after stating that the world we inhabit was at first fluid, and that highly crystalline rocks were deposited before animal or vegetable life began, has demonstrated, that then came the lowest orders of zoophytes and of vegetables, next fishes and reptiles, and trees in vast forests, giving origin to our present beds of coal, then quadrupeds and birds, and shells and plants, *resembling* those of the present æra, but all of which, as species, have utterly perished from the earth; next came alluvial rocks, containing bones of mammoths, &c., and last of all came man. (Cuvier's Preface to his Ossemens Fossiles, and papers by Dr. Fleming in Chalmers' Journal.) This shows that destruction of vegetable and animal life were institutions of nature before man became an inhabitant of the globe. It is beyond the compass of philosophy to explain *why* the world was so constituted. I therefore make no inquiry *why* death was instituted, and refer, of course, only to the dissolution of organized bodies, and not at all to the state of the soul or mind after its separation from the body. These belong to Revelation.

Let us first view the dissolution of the body abstractedly from personal considerations, as a mere natural arrangement. Death, then, appears to be a result of the constitution of all organized beings; for the very definition of the genus, is, that the individuals grow, attain maturity, decay, and die. The human imagination cannot conceive how the former part of this series of movements could exist without the latter, as long as space is necessary to corporeal existence. If all the vegetable and animal productions of nature, from creation downwards, had grown, attained maturity, and there remained, this world would not have been capable of containing one thousandth part of them; so that, on this earth, decaying and dying appear indispensably necessary to admit of reproduction and growth. Viewed abstractedly, then, organized beings live as long as health and vigour continue; but they are subjected to a process of decay, which impairs gradually all their functions, and at last terminates in their dissolution. Now, in the vegetable world, the effect of this law, is, to surround us with young forests, in place of the monotony of everlasting stately full grown woods, standing forth in awful endless majesty, without variation in leaf or bough;—with the vernal bloom of the meadows, changing gracefully into the vigour of summer, and the maturity of autumn;—with the rose, first simply and delicately budding, next fresh and lovely in its blow, and then rich and luxuriant in its perfect condition. In short, when we advert to the law of death, as instituted in the vegetable organized kingdom, and as related to our own faculties of Ideality, Wonder, &c., which desire and delight in the very changes which death introduces, we without hesitation exclaim, that all is wisely, admirably, and wonderfully made. Turning, again, to the animal kingdom, the same fundamental principle prevails. Death removes the old, the worn out, and decayed, and, in their place, the organic law introduces the young, the gay, and the vigorous, to tread the stage with increased agility and delight.

This transfer of existence may readily be granted to be beneficial to the young; but, at first sight, it appears the opposite of benevolent to the old. To have lived at all, is felt as giving a right to continue to live; and the question arises, how can the institution of death, as the result of the organic law, be reconciled with Benevolence and Justice?

In treating of the supremacy of the sentiments, I pointed out, that the grand distinction between them and the propensities, consist in this, that the former are disinterested, generous, and fond of the general good, and the latter altogether selfish in their desires. It is obvious, that death, as an institution of the Creator, must affect these two classes of faculties in the most different manner. The propensities, being confined in their gratification to self, and having no reference to the welfare of any other creature, a being endowed only with them and reflecting intellect, and enabled, by the latter, to discover death and its consequences, would regard it as the most appalling of visitations, and would see in it only utter extinction of all enjoyment. The lower animals, then, whose whole being is composed of the inferior propensities, and several *knowing* faculties, would see death, if they could at all anticipate it, only in this light. So tremendously fearful would it appear to them, as the extinguisher of every pleasure which they had ever felt or could conceive, that we may safely predicate, that the bare prospect of it would render their lives wretched, and that nothing could compensate the agonies of terror, with which an habitual consciousness of it would inspire them. But, by depriving them of *reflecting* organs, the Creator has kindly and effectually preserved them from the influence of this evil. He has thereby rendered them completely blind to its existence. There is not the least reason to believe, that any one of the lower animals, while in health and vigour, has the slightest conception that it is a mortal creature, any more than a tree has that it will die. In consequence, it lives in as full enjoyment of the present, as if it were assured of every agreeable sensation being eternal. Death always takes the individual by surprise, whether it comes in the form of violence, suppressing life in youth, or of slow decay by age; therefore, it really operates in their case as a transference of existence from one being to another, without consciousness of the loss in the one which dies. Let us, however, trace the operation of death, in regard to the lower animals, a little more in detail.

It will not be disputed, that the world is calculated to contain and support only a definite number of living creatures, that the lower animals have received from nature powers of reproduction far beyond what is necessary to supply the waste of life, by natural decay, and that they do not possess intellect sufficient to restrain their numbers within the limits of their means of subsistence. Here, therefore, is an institution in which destruction of life, to a great extent, is necessarily implied. Philosophy cannot tell why death was instituted at first, but, according to the views maintained in this Essay, we should expect to find it connected with, and regulated by, benevolence and justice; that is to say, that it should not be inflicted for the sole purpose of extinguishing the life of individuals, to their damage, without any other result; but that the general system under which it takes place should be, on the whole, favourable to the enjoyment of the race; and this accordingly is the fact. Violent death, and the devouring of one animal by another, are not purely benevolent, because pure benevolence would never inflict pain; but they are instances of destruction guided by benevolence; that is, wherever death proceeds under the institutions of nature, it is accompanied with enjoyment or beneficial consequences to one set of animals or another. Herbivorous animals are exceedingly prolific, yet the supply of vegetable food is limited. Hence, after multiplying for a few years, extensive starvation, the most painful and lingering of all deaths, and the most detrimental to the race, would inevitably ensue; but carnivorous animals have been instituted who kill and eat them; and by this means not only do carnivorous animals reap the pleasures of life, but the numbers of the herbivorous are restrained within such limits, that the individuals among them enjoy existence while they live. The destroyers, again, are limited in their turn. The moment they become too numerous, and carry their devastations too far, their food fails them, and, in their conflicts for the supplies that remain, they extinguish each other, or die of starvation. Nature seems averse from inflicting death extensively by starvation, probably because it impairs the constitution long before it extinguishes life, and has the tendency to produce degeneracy in the race. It may be remarked, also, speculatively, that herbivorous animals must have existed in considerable numbers before the carnivorous began to exercise their functions; for many of the former must die, that one of the latter may live; if a single sheep and a single tiger had been placed together at first, the tiger would have eaten up the sheep at a few meals, and died itself of starvation, in a brief space afterwards. In natural decay, the organs are worn out by mere age, and the animal sinks into gradual insensibility, unconscious that dissolution awaits it. Further, the wolf, the tiger, the lion, and other beasts of prey, instituted by the Creator as instruments of violent death, are provided, in addition to Destructiveness, with large organs of Cautiousness and Secretiveness, that prompt them to steal upon their victims with the unexpected suddenness of a mandate of annihilation, and they are impelled also to inflict death in the most instantaneous and least painful method; the tiger and lion spring from their cover with the rapidity of a thunderbolt, and one blow of their tremendous paws, inflicted at the junction of the head with the neck, produces instantaneous death. The eagle is taught to strike its sharp beak into the spine of the birds which it devours, and their agony endures scarcely for an instant. It has been objected, that the cat plays with the unhappy mouse, and prolongs its tortures; but the cat that does so, is the pampered and well fed inhabitant of a kitchen; the cat of nature is too eager to devour, to indulge in such luxurious gratifications of Destructiveness and Secretiveness. It kills in a moment, and eats. Here, then, is actually a regularly organized process for withdrawing individuals of the lower animals from existence, almost by a fiat of destruction, and thereby making way for a succession of other occupants.

Man is not so merciful towards the lower creatures: but he might be so. Suppose the sheep in the hands of man were to be guillotined, and not maltreated before its execution, the creature would never know that it had ceased to live. And, by the law which I have already explained, man does not with impunity add one unnecessary pang to the death of the lower animals. In the brutal butcher who inflicts torments on calves, sheep, and cattle, while driving them to the slaughter, and who puts them to death in the way supposed to be most conducive to the gratification of his Acquisitiveness, such as bleeding them to death, by successive stages, prolonged for days, to whiten their flesh, —the animal faculties of Destructiveness, Acquisitiveness, Self-esteem, &c., predominate so decidedly in activity, over the moral and intellectual powers, that he is necessarily excluded from all the enjoyments attendant on the supremacy of the human faculties; he, besides, goes into society under the influence of the same base combination, and suffers at every hand animal retaliation, so that he does not escape with impunity for his outrages against the moral law. Here, then, we can perceive nothing malevolent in the institution of death, in so far as regards the lower animals. A pang certainly does attend it; but while Destructiveness must be recognised in the pain, Benevolence is equally perceptible in its effects.

I mentioned formerly, that the organic law rises above the physical, and the moral and intellectual law above the organic; and the present occasion affords an additional illustration of this fact. Under the physical law, no remedial process is instituted to arrest, or restore, against the consequences of infringement. If a mirror falls, and is smashed, by the physical law it remains ever after in fragments; if a ship sinks, it lies still at the bottom of the ocean, chained down by the law of gravitation. Under the organic law, on the other hand, a distinct remedial process is established. If a tree is blown over, every root that remains in the ground will double its exertions to preserve life; if a branch is lopped off, new branches will shoot out in its place; if a leg in an animal is broken, the bone will

reunite; if a muscle is severed, it will grow together; if
an artery is obliterated, the neighbouring arteries will en·
large their dimensions, and perform its functions. The
Creator, however, not to encourage animals to abuse this
benevolent institution, has established pain as an attendant
on infringement of the organic law, and made them suffer
for the violation of it, even while he restores them. It is
under this law that death has received its organic pangs.
Instant death is not attended with pain of any perceptible
duration; and it is only when a lingering death occurs in
youth and middle age, that the suffering is severe; dissolution, however, does not occur at these periods *as a direct
and intentional result of the organic laws*, but as the consequence of infringement of them under the fair and legitimate operation of these laws, the individual whose constitution was at first sound, and whose life has been in accordance with their dictates, lives till old age fairly wears
out his orgnaized frame, and then the pang of expiration is
little perceptible.* The pains of premature death, then,
are the punishments of infringement of the organic law,
and the object of that chastisement probably is to impress

---

* The following table is copied from an interesting article by Mr.
William Fraser, on the History and Constitution of Benefit or Friendly
Societies, published in the Edinburgh New Philosophical Journal for
October, 1827, and is deduced from Returns by Friendly Societies in
Scotland for various years, from 1750 to 1821. It shows how much sick-
ness is dependent on age.

Average Sickness for each Individual.

	Age.	Weeks and Decimals.	Weeks.	Days.	Hours.	Proportion of Sick Members.
Under	20	0.3797	0	2	16	1 in 136.95
	20—30	0.5916	0	4	3	1 " 87.89
	30—40	0.6865	0	4	19	1 " 75.74
	40—50	1.0273	1	0	4	1 " 50.61
	50—60	1.8806	1	6	3	1 " 27.65
	60—70	5.6337	5	4	10	1 " 9.28
Above	70	16.5417	16	3	19	1 " 3.14

upon us the necessity of obeying them that we may live, and to prevent our abusing the remedial process inherent to a great extent in our constitution.

Let us now view death as an institution appointed to man. If it be true, that the organic constitution of man, when sound in its elements, and preserved in accordance with the organic laws, is fairly calculated to endure in health from infancy to old age, and that death when it occurs during the early or middle periods of life, is the consequences of departures from the physical and organic laws, it follows, that, even in premature death, a benevolent principle is discernible. Although the remedial process restores animals from moderate injuries, yet the very nature of the organic law must place a limit to it. If life had been preserved, and health restored, after the brain had been blown to atoms, by a bomb shell, as effectually as a leg that is broken, and a finger that is cut are healed, this would have been an actual abrogation of the organic law; and all the curbs which that law imposes on the lower propensities, and all the incitements which the observance of it affords to the higher sentiments, and intellect, would have been lost. The limit, then, is this; that any departure from the law against which restoration is permitted, shall be moderate in extent, and shall not involve, to a great degree, any organ essential to life, such as the brain, the lungs, the stomach, or intestines. The very maintenance of the law, with all its advantages, requires that restoration from grievous derangement of these organs should not be permitted. When we reflect on the hereditary transmission of qualities to children, we clearly perceive benevolence to the race in the institution, which cuts short the life of an individual in whose person essential organs are so deeply diseased by departures from the organic law, as to be beyond the limits of the remedial process; for the extension of the punishment of his errors over an innumerable posterity is thereby prevented. In premature death, then, we see two objects accomplished ; first, the individual sufferer is withdrawn from agonies which could serve no beneficial end to himself ; he has transgressed the limits of recovery, and prolonged life would be protracted misery ; secondly, the race is guaranteed from the future transmission of his disease by hereditary descent.

The disciple of Mr. Owen, formerly alluded to, who had grievously transgressed the organic law, and suffered a punishment of equal intensity, observed, when in the midst of his agony,—' Philosophers have urged the institution of death, as an argument against divine goodness, but not one of them could experience, for five minutes, the pain which I now endure, without looking upon it as a most merciful arrangement. I have departed from the natural institutions, and suffer the punishment ; but, in death, I see only the Creator's benevolent hand, stretched out to terminate my agonies, when they cease to serve any beneficial end.' On this principle, the death of a feeble and sickly child is an act of mercy to it. It withdraws a being, in whose person the organic laws have been violated, from useless suffering ; cutting short, thereby, also, the transmission of its imperfections to posterity. If, then, the organic institutions which inflict pain and disease as punishments for transgressing them, are founded in benevolence and wisdom ; and, if death, in the early and middle periods of life, is an arrangement for withdrawing the transgressor from further suffering, after return to obedience is impossible, and protecting the race from the consequences of his errors, it also is in itself wise and benevolent.

This, then, leaves us only death in old age as a natural and unavoidable institution of the Creator. It will not be denied, that, if old persons, when their powers of enjoyment are fairly exhausted, and their cup of pleasure full, could be removed from this world, as we have supposed the lower animals to be, in an instant, and without pain or consciousness, to make way for a fresh and vigorous offspring, about to run the career which the old have terminated, there would be no lack of benevolence and justice in the arrangement. At present, while we live in habitual ignorance and neglect of the organic institutions, death probably comes upon us with more pain and agony, even in advanced life, than might be its legitimate accompaniment, if we placed ourselves in accordance with these ; so that we are not now in a condition to ascertain the natural quantum of pain necessarily attendant on death. Judging from analogy, we may conclude, that the close of a long life, founded at first, and afterwards spent, in accordance with the Creator's laws, would not be accompanied with great organic suffering, but that an insensible decay would steal upon the senses. Be this, however, as it may, I observe, in the next place, that as the Creator has bestowed on man animal faculties that fear death, and reason that carries home to him the conviction that he must die, it is an interesting inquiry, Whether he has provided any *natural* means of relief, from the consequences of this combination of terrors ? He has bestowed moral sentiments on man, and arranged the whole of his existence on the principles of their supremacy ; and these, when duly cultivated and enlightened, are calculated to withdraw from him the terrors of death, in the same manner as unconsciousness of its existence saves the lower animals from its horrors.

In regard to the lower animals killed by violence, if reason sees, on the one hand, a momentary pang in parting with life, it perceives the continued existence and enjoyment of beasts of prey, as an advantage attending it on the other, so that every animal that is devoured ministers to the continued life of another. The process is still one of a transfer of existence.

In regard to man, again, the moral sentiments and intellect perceive,

1st. That Amativeness, Philoprogenitiveness, and Adhesiveness, are provided with direct objects of gratification in consequence of the institution of death. If the same individuals had lived here forever, there would have been no field for the enjoyment that flows from the domestic union, and the rearing of offspring. The very institution of these propensities prove, that producing and rearing young, form part of the design of creation; and the successive production of young appears necessarily to imply removal of the old.

2dly. All the other faculties would have been limited in their gratifications. Conceive, for a moment, how much exercise is afforded to our intellectual and moral powers, in acquiring knowledge, communicating it to the young, and in providing for their enjoyments; also, what a delightful exercise of the higher sentiments is implied in the intercourse between the aged and the young; all which pleasures would have been unknown, if there had been no young in existence, which there could not have been, without a succession of individuals.

3dly. Constituted as man is, the succession of individuals withdraws beings whose physical and mental constitutions have run their course, and become impaired in sensibility, and substitutes, in their place, fresh and vigorous minds and bodies, far better adapted for the enjoyment of creation.

4thly. If I am right in the position, that the organic laws transmit, in an increasing ratio, the qualities most active in the parents to their offspring, the law of succession provides for a far higher degree of improvement in the race than could ever have been reached by the permanency of a single generation.

Let us inquire, then, how the moral sentiments are affected by death in old age, as a natural institution.

Benevolence, glowing with a disinterested desire for the diffusion and boundless increase of enjoyment, utters no complaint against death in old age, as a transference of existence from a being impaired in its capacity for usefulness and pleasure, to one fresh and vigorous in all its powers, and fitted to carry forward, to a higher point of improvement, every beneficial measure previously begun. Conscientiousness, if thoroughly enlightened, perceives no infringement of justice in a guest, satiated with enjoyment, being called on to retire from the banquet, to permit a stranger with a keener and more youthful appetite to partake; and Veneration, when instructed by intellect that this is the institution of the Creator, and made acquainted with its objects, bows in humble acquiescence to the law. Now, if these powers have acquired, in any individual, that complete supremacy which they are clearly intended to hold, he will be placed by them as much above the terror of death as a natural institution, as the lower animals are, by being ignorant of its existence. And unless the case were so, man would, by the very knowledge of death, be rendered, during his whole life, more miserable than they.

In these observations, I have said nothing of the prospects of a future existence as a palliative of the evils of dissolution, because I was bound to regard death, in the first instance, as the result of the organic law, and to treat of it as such. But no one who considers that the prospects of a life to come, are directly addressed to Veneration, Hope, Benevolence, and Intellect, can fail to perceive that this consolation also is clearly founded on the principle, that supremacy in the sentiments is intended by the Creator to protect man from its terrors.

The true view of death, then, as a natural institution, is, that it is an essential part of the very system of organization; that birth, growing, and arriving at maturity, as completely imply decay, and death in old age, as morning and noon imply evening and night, as spring and summer imply harvest, or as the source of a river implies a termination of it. Besides, organized beings are constituted by the Creator to be the food of other organized beings, so that some must die that others may live. Man, for instance, cannot live on stones, or earth, or water, which are not organized, but on vegetable and animal substances; so that death is as much, and as essentially, an inherent part of organization as life itself. If vegetables, animals, and men, had been destined for a duration like that of the mountains,—instead of creating a primitive pair of each, and endowing these with extensive powers of reproduction, so as to usher into existence young beings to grow up to maturity by insensible degrees, we may presume, from analogy, that the Creator would have furnished the world with its definite complement of living beings, perfect at first in all their parts and functions, and that these would have remained, like hills, without diminution, and without increase.

To prevent, then, all chance of being misapprehended, I repeat, that I do not at all allude to the state of the soul or mind, after death, but merely to the dissolution of organized bodies; that, according to the soundest view which I am able to obtain of the natural law, pain and death in youth and middle age, in the human species, are consequences of departure from the Creator's laws; while death in old age, by insensible decay, is an essential and apparently indispensable part of the system of organized existence; that this arrangement admits of the succession of individuals, substituting the young and vigorous for the feeble and decayed; that it is directly the means by which organized beings live, and indirectly the means by which Amativeness, Philoprogenitiveness, and a variety of our other faculties obtain gratification; that it admits of the race ascending to a great extent in the scale of improvement, both in their organic and mental qualities; that the moral sentiments, when supreme in activity, and enlightened by intellect, so as to perceive its design and consequences are calculated to place man in harmony with it; while religion addresses its consolation to the same faculties, and completes what reason leaves undone.

If the views now unfolded be correct, death, in old age, will never be abolished, as long as man continues an organized being; but pain and premature death will constantly decrease, in the exact ratio of his obedience to the physical and organic laws. It is interesting to observe, that there is already some evidence of this process being actually in progress. About seventy years ago, tables of the average duration of life, in England, were compiled for the use of the Life Insurance Companies; and from them it appears, that the average of life was then twenty-eight years; that is, 1000 persons being born, and the years which each of them lived being added together, and divided by 1000, gave twentyeight to each. By recent tables, it appears that the average is now thirtytwo years to each; that is to say, by superior morality, cleanliness, knowledge, and general obedience to the Creator's institutions, fewer individuals now perish in infancy, youth, and middle age, than did seventy years ago. Some persons have said, that the difference arises from errors in compiling the old tables, and that the superior habits of the people are not the cause. It is probable, however, that there may be a portion of truth in both views. There may be some errors in the old tables, but it is quite natural that increasing knowledge and stricter obedience to the organic laws, should diminish the number of premature deaths. If this idea be correct, the average duration of life should go on increasing; and our successors, two centuries hence, may probably attain to an average of forty years, and then ascribe to errors in our tables our low average of thirty-two.*

---

* While the above paragraph was in the press, an interesting article on the 'Diminished Mortality in England,' appeared in the Scotsman newspaper, of 16th April, 1828. It coincides with the views of the text; and, as it proceeds on scientific data, it is printed in the Appendix. No. III.

SECTION III.

CALAMITIES ARISING FROM INFRINGMENT OF THE MORAL LAW.

We come now to consider the Moral Law, which is proclaimed by the higher sentiments and intellect acting harmoniously, and holding the animal propensities in subjection. In surveying the moral and religious codes of diferent nations, and the moral and religious opinions of different philosophers, every reflecting mind must have been struck with their diversity. Phrenology, by demonstrating the differences of combination in their faculties, enables us to account for these varieties of sentiment. The code of morality framed by a legislator, in whom Destructiveness, Secretiveness, Acquisitiveness, and Self-esteem were large, and Conscientiousness, Benovolence, and Veneration small, would be very different from one instituted by another lawgiver, in whom this combination was reversed. In like manner, a system of religion, founded by an individual, in whom Destructiveness, Wonder, and Cautiousness were very large, and Veneration, Benevolence, and Conscientiousness deficient, would present views of the Supreme Being widely dissimilar to those which would be promulgated by a person in whom the last three faculties and intellect decidedly predominated. Phrenology shows, that the particular code of morality and religion, *which is most completely in harmony with the whole faculties of the individual,* will necessarily appear to him to be the best, *while he refers only to the dictates of his individual mind, as the standard of right and wrong.* But if we are able to show, that the *whole scheme of external creation is arranged in harmony with certain principles, in preference to others,* so that enjoyment flows upon the individual from without, when his conduct is in conformity with them, and that evil overtakes him when he departs from them, we shall then obviously prove, that the former is the morality and religion established by the Creator; and that individual men, who support different codes, must necessarily be deluded by imperfections in their own minds. That constitution of mind, also, may be pronounced to be the best, which harmonizes most completely with the morality and religion established by the Creator's arrangements. In this view, *morality becomes a science,* and departures from its dictates may be demonstrated as practical follies, injurious to the real interest and happiness of the individual, just as errors in logic are capable of refutation to the understanding. Before we can be in a condition to perceive this, it is obvious that we must know, first, The nature of man, physical, animal, moral, and intellectual; secondly, The relations of the different parts of that nature to each other; and, thirdly, The relationship of the whole to God and external objects. The present Essay is an attempt, (a very feeble and imperfect one indeed,) to arrive, by the aid of phrenology, at a demonstration of morality as a science. The interests dealt with in the investigation are so elevating, and the effort itself is so delightful, that the attempt carries its own reward, however unsuccessful in its own results.

Assuming, then, that, among the faculties of the mind, the higher sentiments and intellect hold the natural supremacy, I shall endeavour to show, that obedience to the dictates of these powers is rewarded with pleasing emotions in the mental faculties themselves, and with the most beneficial external consequences; whereas disobedience is followed by deprivation of these emotions, by painful feelings within the mind, and great external evil.

First. Obedience is attended by pleasing emotions in the faculties. It is scarcely necessary to dwell on the circumstance, that every propensity, sentiment, and intellectual faculty, when gratified in harmony with all the rest, is a fountain of pleasure. How many exquisite thrills of joy arise from Philoprogenitiveness, Adhesiveness, Acquisitiveness, Constructiveness, Love of Approbation, and Self-esteem, when gratified in accordance with the moral sentiments; who that has ever poured forth the aspirations of Hope, Ideality, Wonder, and Veneration, directed to an object in whom Intellect and Conscientiousness also rejoiced, has not experienced the deep delight of such an exercise? Or, who is a stranger to the grateful pleasures attending an active Benevolence? Turning to the intellect, again, what pleasures are afforded by the scenery of nature, by painting, poetry, and music, to those who possess the combination of faculties related to those studies? And how rich a feast does not philosophy yield to those who possess high reflecting organs, combined with Concentrativeness and Conscientiousness? The reader is requested, therefore, to keep steadily in view, that these exquisite rewards are attached by the Creator to the active exercise of our faculties, in accordance with the moral law; and that one punishment, clear, obvious and undeniable, inflicted on those who neglect or infringe the law, is *deprivation* of these pleasures. This is a consideration very little attended to; because mankind, in general, live in such habitual neglect of the moral law, that they have, to a very partial extent, experienced its rewards, and do not know the enjoyment they are deprived of by its infringement. Before its full measure can be judged of, the mind must be instructed in its own constitution, in that of external objects, and in the relationship established between it and them, and between it and the Creator. Until a tolerably distinct perception of these truths is obtained, the faculties cannot enjoy repose, nor act in full vigour or harmony: while, for example, our forefather's regarded the marsh fevers, to which they were subjected, from deficient draining of their fields, and the outrages on person and property, attendant on the wars waged by the English against the Scots, or by one feudal lord against another, even on their own soil, not as punishments for particular infringements of the organic and moral laws, to be removed by obedience to these laws, but as inscrutable dispensations of God's providence, which it behoved them meekly to endure, but not to avert,—so long as such notions were entertained, the full enjoyment which the moral and intellectual faculties were fairly calculated by the Creator to afford, could not be experienced. Benevolence would pine in dissatisfaction ; Veneration would flag in its devotions, and Conscientiousness would suggest endless surmises of disorder and injustice in a scheme of creation, under which such evils occurred, and were left without a remedy ; the full tide of moral, religious, and intellectual enjoyment could not possibly flow, until views, more in accordance with the constitution and desires of the moral faculties were obtained. The same evil afflicts mankind still to a prodigious extent. How is it possible for the Hindoo, Mussulman, Chinese, or the native American, while they continue to worship deities, whose qualities outrage Benevolence, Veneration, and Conscientiousness,—and remain in profound ignorance of almost all the Creator's natural institutions, in consequence of infringing which they suffer punishment without ceasing, to form even a conception of the gratifications which the moral and intellectual nature of man is calculated to enjoy, when exercised in harmony with the Creator's real character and institutions ? This operation of the moral law is not the less real, because many do not recognize it. Sight is not a less excellent gift to those who see, because some men born blind have no conception of the extent of pleasure and advantage from which the want of it cuts them off.

The qualities manifested by the Creator may be inferred from the works of creation ; but it is obvious, that, to arrive at the soundest views, we would require to know his institutions thoroughly. To a grossly ignorant people, who suffer hardly from transgression of his laws, the Deity will appear infinitely more severe and mysterious than to an enlightened nation who know them, avoid the penalties of infringement, and trace the principles of his government through many parts of his works. The character of the Divine Being, under the natural system, will thus go on rising in exact proportion as his works shall be understood. The low and miserable conceptions of God formed by the vulgar Greeks and Romans, were the reflections of their own ignorance of natural, moral, and political science. The discovery and improvement of phrenology must necessarily have a great effect on natural religion. Before phrenology was known, the moral and intellectual constitution of man was unascertained ;—in consequence, the relations of external nature towards it could not be competently judged of; and, while these were involved in obscurity, many of the ways of Providence must have appeared mysterious and severe, which in themselves are quite the reverse. Again, as bodily suffering and mental perplexity would bear a proportion to this ignorance, the character of God would appear to the natural eye in that condition, much more unfavourable than it will do after these clouds of darkness shall have passed away.

Some persons, in their great concernment about a future life, are liable to overlook the practical direction of the mind in the present. When we consider the nature and objects of the mental faculties, we perceive that a great number of them have the most obvious and undeniable reference to this life ; for example, Amativeness, Philoprogenitiveness, Combativeness, Destructiveness, Acquisitiveness, Secretiveness, Cautiousness, Self-esteem, and Love of Approbation, with Size, Form, Colour, Weight, Tune, Wit, and probably other faculties, stand in such evident relationship to this particular world, with its moral and physical arrangements, that if they were not capable of legitimate application here, it would be difficult to assign a reason for their being bestowed on us. We possess also Benevolence, Veneration, Hope, Ideality, Wonder, Conscientiousness, and reflecting Intellect, all of which appear to be particularly adapted to a higher sphere. But the important consideration is, that here on earth these two sets of faculties are combined; and on the same principle that led Sir Isaac Newton to infer the combustibility of the diamond, I am disposed to expect that the external world, when its constitution and relations shall be sufficiently understood, will be found to be in harmony with all our faculties, and of course that the character of the Deity, as unfolded by the works of creation, will more and more gratify our moral and intellectual powers, in proportion as knowledge advances. The structure of the eye is admirably adapted to the laws of light; that of the ear to the laws of sound; that of the muscles to the laws of gravitation; and it would be strange if our mental constitution was not as wisely adapted to the general order of the external world.

This principle, then, is universal, and admits of no exception, That inactivity and want of power, in every faculty, is attended with deprivation of the pleasures attendant on its vivacious exercise. He who is so deficient in Tune that he cannot distinguish melody, is cut off from a vast source of gratification enjoyed by him who possesses that organ vigorous and highly cultivated; and the same principle holds in the case of every other organ and faculty. Criminals and profligates of every description, therefore, from the very constitution of human nature, are excluded from great enjoyments attending virtue; and this is the first natural punishment to which they are inevitably liable. Persons also, who are ignorant of the constitutions of their own minds, and the relations between external objects, not only suffer many direct evils on this account; but, through the consequent inactivity of their faculties, are besides, deprived of many exalted enjoyments. The works of creation, and the character of the Deity, are the legitimate objects of our highest powers; and hence he who is blind to their qualities loses nearly the whole benefit of his moral and intellectual existence. If there is any one to whom these gratifications are unknown, or appear trivial, he must either, to a very considerable degree, be still under the dominion of the animal propensities, or his views of the Creator's character and institutions, must not be in harmony with the natural dictates of the moral sentiments and intellect.

But, in the second place, as the world is arranged on the principle of the supremacy of the moral sentiments and intellect, observance of the moral law is attended with external advantages, and infringement of it with positive evil consequences; and, from this constitution, arises the second natural punishment of misconduct.

Let us trace the advantages of obedience.—In the domestic circle; if we preserve habitually Benevolence, Conscientiousness, Veneration, and Intellect supreme, it is quite undeniable, that we shall raise the moral and intellectual faculties of children, servants, and assistants, to love us, and to yield us willing service, obedience, and aid. Our commands will then be reasonable, mild, and easily executed, and the commerce will be that of love. With our equals, again, in society, what would we not give for a friend in whom we were perfectly convinced of the supremacy of the sentiments; what love, confidence, and delight, would we not repose in him? To a merchant, physician, lawyer, magistrate, or an individual in any public employment, how invaluable would be the habitual supremacy of the sentiment? The Creator has given different talents to different individuals, and limited our powers, so that we execute any work best by confining our attention to one department of labour,—an arrangement which amounts to a direct institution of separate trades and professions. Under the natural laws, then, the manufacturer may pursue his calling with the entire approbation of all the moral sentiments, for he is dedicating his talents to supply the wants of his fellow men ; and how much more successful will he not be, if his every wish is accompanied by the desire to act benevolently and honestly towards those who are to consume and pay for the products of his labour? He cannot gratify his Acquisitiveness half so successfully by any other method. The same remark applies to the merchant, the lawyer, and physician. The lawyer and physician, whose whole spirits breathe a disinterested desire to consult, as a paramount object, the best interests of their clients and patients, not only obtain the direct reward of gratifying their own moral faculties, which is no slight enjoyment, but they reap a positive gratification to their Self-esteem and Love of Approbation, in a high and well founded reputation, and to their Acquisitiveness, in increasing emolument, not grudgingly paid, but willingly offered, from minds that feel the worth of the services bestowed.

There are three conditions required by the moral and intellectual law, which must all be observed to ensure its rewards ; 1st. The department of industry selected must be really useful to human beings : Benevolence demands this ; 2dly. The quantum of labour bestowed must bear a just proportion to the natural demand for the commodity produced ; Intellect requires this ; and, 3dly. In our social connexions, we must imperatively attend to the organic law, that different individuals possess different developements of the brain, and in consequence different natural talents and dispositions, and we must rely on each only to the extent warranted by his natural endowment.

If, then, an individual has received, at birth, a sound organic constitution, and favourably developed brain, and if he live in accordance with the physical, the organic, the moral, and intellectual laws, it appears to me that, in the constitution of the world, he has received an assurance from the Creator, of provision for his animal wants, and a high enjoyment in the legitimate exercise of his various mental powers.

I have already observed, that, before we can obey the Creator's institutions, we must know them, and that the science which teaches the physical laws is natural philosophy; that the organic laws belong to the department of anatomy and physiology; and I now add, that it is the business of the political economists to unfold the kinds of industry that are really necessary to the welfare of mankind, and the degrees of labour that will meet with a just reward. The leading object of political economy, as a science, is to increase enjoyment, by directing the application of industry. To attain this end, however, it is obviously necessary that the nature of man,—the constitution of the physical world,—and the relations between these, should be known. Hitherto, the knowledge of the first of these elementary parts has been very deficient, and, in consequence, the whole superstructure has been weak and unproductive, in comparison of what it may become, when founded on a more perfect basis. Political economists have never dreamt, that the world is arranged on the principle of supremacy of the moral sentiments and intellect; and, consequently, that, to render man happy, *his leading pursuits must be such as will exercise and gratify these powers*, and that his life will necessarily be miserable, if devoted entirely to the production of wealth. They have proceeded on the notion, that the accumulation of wealth is the *summum bonum;* but all history teaches, that national happiness does not increase in proportion to national riches; and until they shall perceive and teach, that intelligence and morality are the foundation of all lasting prosperity, they will never interest the great body of mankind, nor give a valuable direction to their efforts.

If the views contained in the present Essay be sound, it will become a leading object with future masters in that science, to demonstrate the necessity of civilized man limiting his physical, and increasing his moral and intellectual occupations, as the only means of saving himself from ceaseless punishment under the natural laws.

The idea of men, in general, being taught natural philosophy, anatomy, and physiology, political economy, and the other sciences that expound the natural laws, has been sneered at, as utterly absurd and ridiculous. But I would ask, in what occupations are human beings so urgently engaged, that they *have no leisure* to bestow on the study of the Creator's laws? A course of natural philosophy would occupy sixty or seventy hours in the delivery; a course of anatomy and physiology the same; and a course of phrenology can be delivered pretty fully in forty hours! These, twice or thrice repeated, would serve to initiate the student so that he could afterwards advance in the same paths, by the aid of observation and books. Is life, then, so brief, and are our hours so urgently occupied by higher and more important duties, that we cannot afford those pittances of time to learn the laws that regulate our existence! No. The only difficulty is in obtaining the *desire* for the knowledge; in seeing the necessity and advantage of it, and then time will not be wanting. No idea can be more preposterous, than that of human beings having no time to study and obey the natural institutions. These laws punish so severely, when neglected, that they cause the offender to lose tenfold more time in undergoing his chastisement, than would be requisite to obey them. A gentleman extensively engaged in business, whose nervous and digestive systems have been impaired by neglect of the organic laws, was desired to walk in the open air at least one hour a-day; to repose from all exertion, bodily and mental, for one full hour after breakfast, and another full hour after dinner, because the brain cannot expend its energy in thinking and in aiding digestion at the same time; and to practice moderation in diet; which last he regularly observed; but he laughed at the very idea of his having three hours a-day to spare for attention to his health. The reply was, that the organic laws admit of no exception, and that he must either obey them, or take the consequences; but that the time lost by the punishment would be double or treble that requisite for obedience; and, accordingly, the fact was so. Instead of his attending an appointment, it is quite usual for him to send a note, perhaps, at two in the afternoon, in these terms :— I was so distressed with headache last night, that I never closed my eyes, and to-day I am still incapable of being out of bed.' On other occasions, he is out of bed, but apologizes for incapacity to attend to business, on account of an intolerable pain in the region of the stomach. In short, if the hours lost in these painful sufferings were added together, and distributed over the days when he is able for duty, he would find them far outnumber those which would suffice for obedience to the organic laws, and with this difference in the results; by neglect he loses both his hours and his enjoyment; whereas, by obedience, he would be rewarded by aptitude for business, and a pleasing consciousness of existence.

We shall understand the operation of the moral and intellectual laws, however, more completely, by attending to the evils which arise from neglect of them.

As to INDIVIDUALS. At present, the almost universal persuasion of civilized man, is, that happiness consists in the possession of wealth, power, and external splendour; objects related to the animal faculties and intellect much more than to the moral sentiments. In consequence, each individual sets out in the pursuit of these as the chief business of his life; and, in the ardour of the chase, he recognizes no limitations on the means which he may employ, except those imposed by the municipal law. He does not perceive or acknowledge the existence of natural laws, determining not only the sources of his happiness, but the steps by which it may be attained. From this moral and intellectual blindness, merchants and manufacturers, in numberless instances, hasten to be rich beyond the course of nature; that is to say, they engage in enterprises far exceeding the extent of their capital, or capacity; they place their property in the hands of debtors, whose natural talents and morality are so low, that they ought never to have been trusted with a shilling; they send their goods to sea without insuring them, or leave them uninsured in their own warehouses; they ask pecuniary accommodation from other merchants, to enable them to carry on their undue speculations, and become security for them in return, and both fall in consequence of blindly following acquisitiveness to extremities; or they live in splendour and extravagance, far beyond the extent of the natural return of their capital and talents. In every one of these instances, the calamity is obviously the consequence of infringement of the moral and intellectual law. The lawyer, medical practitioner, or probationer in the church, who is disappointed in his reward, will be found erroneously to have placed himself in a profession, for which his natural talents and dispositions did not fit him, or to have pursued his vocation under the guidance chiefly of the lower propensities, prefering selfishness to honourable regard for the interests of his employers. Want of success in these professions, appears to me to be owing, in a high degree, to three causes; first, The brain being too small, or constitutionally lymphatic, so that the mind does not act with sufficient energy to make an impression; secondly, some particular organs indispensably requisite to success, being very deficient, as Language, or Causality, in a lawyer, the first rendering him incapable of ready utterance, and the second destitute of that intuitive sagacity, which sees at a glance the bearing of the facts and principles founded on by his adversary, so as to estimate the just inferences that follow, and to point them out. A lawyer, who is weak in this power, appears to his client like a pilot who does not know the shoals and the rocks.

His deficiency is perceived whenever difficulty presents itself, and he is pronounced unsafe to take charge of great interests; he is then passed by, and suffers the responsibility of an erroneous choice of profession; or, thirdly, Predominance of the animal and selfish faculties. The client and the patient discriminate instinctively between the cold, pithless, but pretending manner of Acquisitiveness and Love of Approbation, and the unpretending, genuine warmth of Benevolence, Veneration, and Conscientiousness; and they discover very speedily that the intellect inspired by the latter sees more clearly, and manages more successfully, their interests, than when animated only by the former; the victim of selfishness either never rises, or sinks, wondering why his merits are neglected.

In all these instances, the failure of the merchant, and the bad success of the lawyer, &c. are the consequences of having infringed the natural laws; so that the evil they suffer is the punishment for having failed in a great duty, not only to society, but to themselves.

The greatest difficulties, however, present themselves, in tracing the operation of the moral and intellectual laws, in the wide field of social life. An individual may be made to comprehend how, if he commits an error, he should suffer a particular punishment; but when calamity overtakes whole classes of the community, each person absolves himself from all share of the blame, and regards himself as simply the victim of a general but inscrutable visitation. Let us, then, examine briefly the Social Law.

In regarding the human faculties, we perceive that numberless gratifications spring from the social state. The muscles of a single individual could not rear the habitations, build the ships, forge the anchors, construct the machinery, or, in short, produce the countless enjoyments that everywhere surround us, in consequence of men being constituted, so as instinctively to combine their powers and skill, to obtain a common end. Here, then, are prodigious advantages resulting directly from the social law; but, in the next place, social intercourse is the means of affording direct gratification to a variety of our mental faculties. If we live in solitude, the propensities of Amativeness, Philoprogenitiveness, Adhesiveness, Love of Approbation, the sentiments of Benevolence, Veneration, Conscientiousness, Wonder, Language, and the reflecting faculties, would be deprived, some of them absolutely, and others of them nearly, of all opportunities of gratification. The social law, then, is the source of the highest delights of our nature, and its institution indicates the greatest benevolence and wisdom towards us, in the Creator.

Still, however, this law does not suspend or subvert the laws instituted for man as an individual. If we imagine an individual to go to sea for his own gratification in a ship, the natural laws require that his intellectual faculties shall be instructed in navigation, also in the nature of the coasts and seas which he traverses; that he shall know and avoid the shoals, currents, and eddies; that he shall trim his canvas in proportion to the gale; and that his animal faculties shall be so much under subjection to his moral sentiments, that he shall not abandon himself to drunkenness, sloth, or any animal indulgence, when the natural laws require him to be watchful at his duty. If he obey the natural laws, he will be safe as an individual; and if he disobey them he will be drowned.* Now, if a crew and passengers desire to avail themselves of the social law, that is, to combine their powers and activity under one leader or chief, by doing which they may sail in a large ship, have ample stores of provisions, divide their labour, enjoy each other's society, &c., and if at the same time they fulfil the moral and intellectual laws, by placing, in the situation of captain, an

---

* I waive at present the question of storms, which he could not foresee, as these fall under the head of ignorance of natural laws, which may be subsequently discovered.

individual fully qualified for that duty, they will enjoy the reward in sailing safely, and in comfort; if they disregard these laws, and place an individual in charge of the ship, whose intellectual faculties are weak, whose animal propensities are strong, whose moral sentiments are in abeyance, and who, in consequence, habitually neglects the natural laws, then they will suffer the penalty in being wrecked.

I know it will be objected that the crew and passengers do not appoint the captain; but, in every case, except impressment in the British navy, they may go in, or stay out, of a particular ship, as they discover the captain to possess the natural qualities or not. This, at present, I am aware, ninety-nine individuals out of the hundred never inquire into; but so do ninety-nine out of the hundred neglect many of the other natural laws, and suffer the penalty, because their moral and intellectual faculties have never yet been instructed in their existence and effects, or trained to observe and obey them. But they have the power from nature of obeying them, if properly taught and trained; and, besides, I give this merely as an illustration of the mode of operation of the social law.

Another example may be given. By employing servants, the labours of life are rendered less burdensome to the master; but he must employ individuals who know the moral law, and who possess the desire to act under it; otherwise, as a punishment for neglecting this requisite, he may be robbed, cheated, or murdered in bed. Phrenology presents the means of observing this law, in a degree quite unattainable without it, by the facility which it affords of discovering the natural talents and dispositions of individuals.

By entering into copartnerships, merchants, and other persons in business, may extend their employment, and gain advantages beyond those they could reap, if labouring as individuals. But, by the natural law, each must take care that his partner knows, and is inclined to obey, the moral and intellectual law, as the only condition on which the Creator will permit him *securely* to reap the *advantages* of the social compact. If a partner in China is deficient in intellect and moral sentiments, another in London may be utterly ruined. It is said that this is the innocent suffering for or along with the guilty; but it is not so. It is an example of a person seeking to obtain the *advantages* of the social law, without conceiving himself bound to obey the conditions required by it; the first of which is, that those individuals, of whose services he avails himself, shall observe the moral and intellectual laws.

Let us now advert to the calamities which overtake whole classes of men, or COMMUNITIES, under the social law, trace their origin, and see how far they are attributable to infringement of the Creator's laws.

If I am right in representing the whole faculties of man as intended by the Creator to be gratified, and the moral sentiments and intellect, as the higher and directing powers, with which all natural institutions are in harmony; it follows, that if large communities of men, in their systematic conduct, habitually seek the gratification of the inferior propensities, and allow either no part, or too small and inadequate a part, of their time to the regular employment of the higher powers, they will act in direct opposition to the natural institutions; and will, of course, suffer the punishment in sorrow and disappointment. Now, to confine ourselves to our own country, it is certain that, until within these few years, the labouring population of Britain were not taught that it was any part of their duty, as rational creatures, to restrain their propensities, so as not to multiply their numbers beyond the demand for their labours, and the supply of food for their offspring; and up to the present hour this most obvious and important doctrine is not admitted by one in a thousand, and not acted upon as a practical principle by one in ten thousand of those whose happiness or misery depends on observance of it. The doctrine of MALTHUS, that 'population cannot go on perpetually increasing, without pressing on the limits of the means of subsistence, and that a check of some kind or other must, sooner or later, be opposed to it,' just amounts to this,—that the means of subsistence are not susceptible of such rapid and unlimited increase as population, and in consequence that the Amative propensity must be restrained by reason, otherwise it will be checked by misery. This principle is in accordance with the views of human nature maintained in this Essay, and applies to all the faculties; thus Philoprogenitiveness, when indulged in opposition to reason leads to spoiling children, which is followed directly by misery both to them and their parents. Acquisitiveness, when uncontrolled by reason, leads to avarice or theft, and these again carry suffering in their train.

But so far from attending to such views, the lives of the inhabitants of Britain generally are devoted to the acquisition of wealth, of power and distinction, or of animal pleasure; in other words, the great object of the labouring classes, is to live and gratify the inferior propensities; of the mercantile and manufacturing population, to gratify Acquisitiveness and Self-esteem; of the more intelligent class of gentlemen, to gratify Self-esteem and Love of Approbation, in political, literary, or philosophical eminence; and of another portion, to gratify Love of Approbation, by supremacy in fashion; and these gratifications are sought by means not in accordance with the dictates of the higher sentiments, but by the joint aid of the intellect and propensities. If the supremacy of moral sentiment and intellect be the natural law, then, as often observed, every circumstance connected with human life must be in harmony with it; that is to say, first, After rational restraint on population, and with the proper use of the machinery, such moderate labour as will leave ample time for the systematic exercise of the higher powers, will suffice to provide for human wants: and, secondly, If this exercise be neglected, and the time which ought to be dedicated to it employed in labour to gratify the propensities, direct evil will ensue; and this accordingly appears to me to be exactly the result.

By means of machinery, and the aids derived from science, the ground can be cultivated, and every imaginable necessary and luxury produced in ample abundance, by a moderate expenditure of labour by any population not in itself superabundant. If men were to stop whenever they had reached this point, and dedicate the residue of each day to moral and intellectual pursuits, the consequence would be, ready and steady because not overstocked, markets. Labour, pursued till it provided abundance, but not redundant superfluity, would meet with a certain and just reward: and would yield also, a vast increase of happiness; for no joy equals that which springs from the moral sentiments and intellect excited by the contemplation, pursuit, and observance, of the Creator's institutions. Further, morality would be improved; for men being happy, would cease to be vicious; and, lastly, There would be improvement in the organic, moral, and intellectual capababilities of the race; for the active, moral and intellectual organs in the parents would increase the volume of these in their offspring; so that each generation would start not only with greater stores of acquired knowledge than their predecessors possessed, but with higher natural capabilities of turning these to account.

Before merchants and manufacturers can be expected to act in this manner, a great change must be effected in their sentiments and perceptions; but so was a striking revolution effected in their ideas and practices of the tenantry west of Edinburgh, when they removed the stagnant pools between each ridge of land, and banished ague from

their district. If any reader will compare the state of
Scotland during the thirteenth, fourteenth, and fifteenth
centuries, correctly and spiritedly represented in Sir
Walter Scott's Tales of a Grandfather, with its present
condition, in regard to knowledge, morality, religion, and
the comparative ascendency of the rational over the animal
part of our nature, he will perceive so great an improvement in later times, that the commencement of the mil-
lennium itself, in five or six hundred years hence, would
scarce be a greater advance beyond the present, than the
present is over the past. If the laws of the Creator be
really what are here represented, and if they were once
taught as elementary truths to every class of the community, and the sentiment of Veneration called in to enforce
obedience to them, a set of new motives and principles
would be brought into play, calculated to accelerate the
change; especially if it were seen, what, in the next place,
I proceed to show, that the consequences of neglecting
these laws are the most serious visitations of suffering that
can well be imagined. The labouring population of
Britain is taxed with exertion for ten, twelve, and some
even fourteen hours a day, exhausting their muscular and
nervous energy, so as utterly to incapacitate them, and
leaving, besides, no leisure, for moral and intellectual pursuits. The consequence of this is, that all markets are
overstocked with produce; prices first fall ruinously low;
the operatives are then thrown idle, and left in destitution
of the necessaries of life, until the surplus produce of their
formerly excessive labours, and perhaps something more,
are consumed; after this takes place, prices rise too high
in consequence of the supply falling rather below the demand; the labourers resume their toil, on their former system of excessive exertion; they again overstock the market, and again are thrown idle, and suffer dreadful misery.

In 1825-6-7 we witnessed this operation of the natural
laws: large bodies of starving and unemployed labourers

were then supported on charity. How many hours did they not stand idle, and how much of excessive toil would not these hours have relieved, if distributed over the periods when they were overworked? The results of that excessive exertion were seen in the form of untenanted houses, of shapeless piles of goods decaying in warehouses, in short, in every form in which misapplied industry could go to ruin. These observations are strikingly illustrated by the following official report, copied from the public newspapers :

'State of the Unemployed Operatives, *resident in Edinburgh*, who are supplied with work by a Committee, constituted for that purpose, according to a list made up on Wednesday, the 14th March, 1827.

'The number of unemployed operatives who have been remitted by the Committee for work, up to the 14th of March are 1481

'And the number of cases they have rejected, after having been particularly investigated, for being bad characters, giving in false statements, or being only a short time out of work, &c. &c. are 446

Making together 1927

'Besides these, several hundreds have been rejected by the Committee, as, from the applicants' *own* statement, they were not considered as cases entitled to receive relief, and were not, therefore, remitted for investigation.

'The wages allowed is 5s. per week, with a peck of meal to those who have families. Some youths are only allowed 3s. of wages.

'The particular occupations of those sent to work are as follows : —242 masons, 634 labourers, 66 joiners, 19 plasterers, 76 sawyers, 19 slaters, 45 smiths, 40 painters, 36 tailors, 55 shoemakers, 20 gardeners, 229 various trades. Total 1481."

Edinburgh is not a manufacturing city, and if so much misery existed in it in proportion to its population, what must have been the condition of Glasgow, Manchester, and other manufacturing towns ?*

---

* In the Appendix, No. IV. several interesting documents are given, in further elucidation of these principles.

Here, then, the Creator's laws show themselves paramount, even when men set themselves systematically to infringe them. He intended the human race, under the moral law, not to pursue Acquisitiveness excessively, but to labour only a certain and a moderate portion of their lives; and although they do their utmost to defeat this intention, they cannot succeed; they are constrained to remain idle as many days and hours, while their surplus produce is consuming, as would have served for the due exercise of their moral and intellectual faculties and the preservation of their health, if they had dedicated them regularly to these ends from day to day, as time passed over their heads. But their punishment proceeds: the extreme exhaustion of nervous and muscular energy, with the absence of all moral and intellectual excitement, create the excessive craving for the stimulus of ardent spirits which distinguishes the labouring population of the present age; this calls into predominant activity the organs of the Animal Propensities, these descend to the children by the law already explained; increased crime, and a deteriorating population, are the results; and a moral and intellectual incapacity for arresting the evils, becomes greater with the lapse of every generation.

According to the principles of the present Essay, what are called by commercial men 'times of prosperity,' are seasons of the greatest infringement of the natural laws, and precursors of great calamities. Times are not reckoned prosperous, unless *all* the industrious population is employed during *the whole day*, hours of eating and sleeping only excepted, in the production of *wealth*. This is a dedication of their whole lives to the service of the propensities, and must necessarily terminate in punishment, if the world is constituted on the principle of supremacy of the higher powers.

This truth has already been illustrated more than once in the history of commerce. The following is a recent example.

By the combination laws, workmen were punishable for uniting to obtain a rise of wages, when an extraordinary demand occurred for their labour. These laws being obviously unjust, were at length repealed. In summer and autumn 1825, however, commercial men conceived themselves to have reached the highest point of prosperity, and the demand for labour was unlimited. The operatives availed themselves of the opportunity to better their condition, formed extensive combinations; and, because their demands were not complied with, struck work, and continued idle for months in succession. The master manufacturers clamored against the new law, and complained that the country would be ruined, if combinations were not again declared illegal, and suppressed by force. According to the principles of this Essay, the just law must from the first have been *the most beneficial for all parties* affected by it; and the result amply confirmed this idea. Subsequent events proved that the extraordinary demand for labourers in 1825 was entirely factitious, fostered by an overwhelming issue of bank paper, much of which ultimately turned out to be worthless; in short, that, during the combinations, the master manufacturers were engaged in an extensive system of speculative over-production, and that the combinations of the workmen presented a *natural check* to this erroneous proceeding. The ruin that overtook the masters in 1826 arose from their having accumulated, under the influence of unbridled Acquisitiveness, vast stores of commodities which were not required by society; and to have compelled the labourers, by force, to manufacture more at their bidding, would obviously have been to aggravate the evil. It is a well known fact, accordingly, that those masters whose operatives most resolutely refused to work, and who, on this account, clamoured loudest against the law, were the greatest gainers in the end. Their stocks of goods were sold off at high prices during the speculative period; and when the revulsion came, instead of being ruined by the fall of property, they were prepared, with their capitals at command, to avail themselves of the depreciation, to make new and highly profitable investments. Here again, therefore, we perceive the law of justice vindicating itself, and benefiting by its operation even those individuals who blindly denounced it as injurious to their interests. A practical faith in the doctrine that the world is arranged by the Creator, in harmony with the moral sentiments and intellect, would be of unspeakable advantage both to rulers and subjects; for they would then be able to pursue with greater confidence the course dictated by moral rectitude, convinced that the result would prove beneficial, even although, when they took the first step, they could not distinctly perceive by what means.

In the whole system of education and treatment of the labouring population, the laws of the Creator, such as I have now endeavoured to expound them, are neglected, and their moral and intellectual cultivation is scarcely known. The Schools of Art, and ' the Library of Useful Knowledge,' are laudable attempts at a better order of things; and I hail with joy their increase; but they too much exclude the science of human nature, and, in consequence, will remain comparatively barren. From indications which already appear, however, I think it probable that the labouring classes will ere long recognise Phrenology, and the natural laws, as deeply interesting to themselves; and whenever their minds shall be opened to rational views of their own constitution as men, and their condition as members of society, I venture to predict that they will devote themselves to improvement with a zeal and earnestness that in a few generations will change the aspect of their class.

The consequences of the present system of departing from the moral law, on the middle orders of the community, are in accordance with its effects on the lower. Uncertain gains, continual fluctuations in fortune, absence of all reliance on moral and intellectual principles in their pursuits, a gambling spirit, an insatiable appetite for wealth, alternately extravagant joys of excessive prosperity and bitter miseries of disappointed ambition, render the whole lives of merchants vanity and vexation of spirit. Nothing is more essential to human happiness than fixed principles of action, on which we can rely for our present safety and future welfare ; and the Creator's laws, when seen and followed, afford this support and delight to our faculties in the highest degree. It is one, not of the least, of the punishments that overtake the middling classes for neglect of these laws, that they do not, as a permanent condition of mind, feel secure and internally at peace with themselves. When the excitement of business has subsided, vacuity and craving are felt within. These proceed from the moral and intellectual faculties calling aloud for exercise ; but, through ignorance of their own nature, fashionable amusements, or intoxicating liquors, are resorted to, and, with these, a vain attempt is made to fill up the void of life. I know that this class ardently desires a change that would remove the miseries described, and will zealously coöperate in the diffusing of knowledge, by which means alone it can be introduced.

The responsibility which overtakes the higher classes is equally obvious. If they do not engage in some active pursuit, so as to give scope to their energies, they suffer the evils of ennui, morbid irritability, and excessive relaxation of the functions of mind and body, which carry in their train more suffering than is entailed even on the operatives by excessive labour. If they pursue ambition in the senate or the field, or in literature or philosophy, their real success is in exact proportion to the approach which they make to observance of the supremacy of the sentiments and intellect. Franklin, Washington, and Bolivar, may be contrasted with Sheridan and Bonaparte, as illustrations.

Sheridan and Napoleon did not, systematically, pursue objects sanctioned by the higher sentiments and intellect, as the end of their exertions ; and no person, who is a judge of human emotions, can read their lives, and consider what must have passed within their minds, without coming to the conclusion, that, even in their most brilliant moments of external prosperity, the canker was gnawing within, and that there was no moral relish of the present, or reliance on the future ; but a mingled tumult of inferior propensities and intellect, carrying with it an habitual feeling of unsatisfied desires.

Let us now consider the effect of the moral law on NATIONAL prosperity.

If the Creator has constituted the world in harmony with the dictates of the higher sentiments, the highest prosperity of each particular nation should be thoroughly compatible with that of every other ; that is to say, England, by sedulously cultivating her own soil, pursuing her own courses of industry, founding her internal institutions and her external relations on the principles of Benevolence, Veneration, and Justice, which imply abstinence from wars of aggression, from conquest, and from all selfish designs of commercial monopoly, would be in the highest condition of prosperity and enjoyment that nature would admit of; and every step that she deviated from these principles, would carry an inevitable punishment along with it. The same statement might be made relative to France and every other nation. According to this principle, also, the Creator should have conferred on each nation some peculiar advantages of soil, climate, situation, or genius, which would enable it to carry on amicable intercourse with its fellow states, in a beneficial exchange of the products peculiar to each ; so that the higher one rose in morality, intelligence, and riches, it ought to become so much the more estimable and valuable as a neighbour to all the surrounding states. This is so obviously the real constitution of nature, that proof of it is superfluous.

England, however, as a nation, has set this law at absolute defiance. She has led the way in taking the propensities as her guides, in founding her laws and institutions on them, and in following them out in her practical conduct. England invented restrictions on trade, and carried them to the greatest height; she conquered colonies, and ruled them in the full spirit of selfishness; she encouraged lotteries and fostered the slave trade, carried paper money and the most avaricious spirit of manufacturing and speculating in commerce to their highest pitch; defended corruption in Parliament, distributed churches and seats on the bench of Justice, on principles purely selfish; all in direct oppostion to the supremacy of the moral law. If the world had been created in harmony with predominance of the animal faculties, England should have been a most felicitous nation; but as the reverse is the case, we should expect a severe national responsibility to flow from these departures from the divine institutions; and grievous accordingly has been, and, I fear, will be, the punishment.

The principle which regulates national responsibility is, that the precise combination of faculties which leads to the national transgression, carries in its train the punishment. Nations are under the moral and intellectual law, as well as individuals. A carter who half starves his horse, and unmercifully beats it, to supply, by the stimulus of pain, the vigour that nature intended to flow from abundance of food, may be supposed to practise this barbarity with impunity in this world, if he evade the eye of Mr. Martin, and that of the police; but this is not the case. The hand of Providence reaches him by a direct punishment: He fails in his object, for blows cannot supply the vigour which, by the constitution of the horse, flows only from sufficiency of wholesome food. In his conduct, he manifests an excessive Combativeness and Destructiveness, with deficient Benevolence, Veneration, Justice, and Intellect, and he cannot reverse this character, by merely averting his eyes and his hand from the horse. He carries these dispositions into the bosom of his family, and into the company of his associates, and a variety of evil consequences ensue. The delights that spring from active moral sentiments and intellectual powers, are necessarily unknown to him; and the difference between these pleasures, and the sensations attendant on his moral and intellectual condition, are as great as between the external splendour of a king and the naked poverty of a beggar. It is true that he has never felt the enjoyment, and does not know the extent of his loss; but still the difference exists; *we* see it, and know that, as a direct consequence of this state of mind, he is excluded from a very great and exalted pleasure. Further; his active animal faculties rouse the Combativeness, Destructiveness, Self-esteem, Secretiveness, and Cautiousness, of his wife, children, and associates, against him, and they inflict on him animal punishment. He, no doubt, goes on to eat, drink, blaspheme, and abuse his horse, day after day, apparently as if Providence approved of his conduct; but he neither feels, nor can any one who attends to his condition believe him to feel, *happy;* he is uneasy, discontented, and disliked,—all which sensations are his punishment, and it is fairly owing to his own grossness and ignorance that he does not connect it with his offence. Let us apply these remarks to nations. England, for instance, under the impulses of an excessively strong Acquisitiveness, Self-esteem, and Destructiveness, for a long time protected the slave trade. Now, according to the law which I am explaining, during the periods of greatest sin in this respect, the same combination of faculties ought to be found working most vigorously in her other institutions, and producing punishment for that offence. There ought to be found in these periods a general spirit of domineering and rapacity in her public men, rendering them little mindful of the welfare of the people; injustice and harshness in her taxations and public laws; and a spirit of aggression and hostility towards other nations, provoking retaliation of her insults. And, accordingly, I have been informed as a matter of fact, that, while these measures of injustice were publicly patronised by the government, its servants vied with each other in injustice towards it, and that its subjects dedicated their talents and enterprise towards corrupting its officers, and cheating it of its due. Every trader who was liable to excise or custom duties, evaded the one-half of them, and felt no disgrace in doing so. A gentleman, who was subject to the excise laws fifty years ago, described to me the condition of his trade at that time. The excise officers, he said, regarded it as an understood matter, that at least one half of the goods manufactured were to be smuggled without being charged with duty; but then, said he, 'they made us pay a moral and pecuniary penalty that was at once galling and debasing. We were required to ask them to our table at all meals, and place them at the head of it in our holiday parties; when they fell into debt, we were obliged to help them out of it; when they moved from one house to another, our servants and carts were in requisition to perform this office; and, by way of keeping up discipline upon us, and also to make a show of duty, they chose every now and then to step in and detect us in a fraud, and get us fined; if we submitted quietly, they told us that they would make us amends, by winking at another fraud; and generally did so; but if our indignation rendered passive obedience impossible, and we spoke our mind of their character and conduct, they enforced the law on *us*, while they relaxed it on our neighbours; and these being rivals in trade, undersold us in the market, carried away our customers, and ruined our business. Nor did the bondage end here. We could not smuggle without the aid of our servants; and as they could, on occasion of any offence given to themselves, carry information to the head quarters of excise, we were slaves to them also, and were obliged tamely to submit to a degree of drunkenness and insolence, that appears to me now perfectly intolerable. Further ; this evasion and oppression did us no good; for all the trade were alike, and we just sold our goods so much cheaper the more duty we evaded; so that our individual success did not depend upon superior skill and superior morality, in making an excellent article at a moderate price, but upon superior capacity for fraud, meanness, sycophancy, and every possible baseness. Our lives were anything but enviable. Conscience, although greatly blunted by practices that were universal, and viewed as inevitable, still whispered that they were wrong; our sentiments of self-respect very frequently revolted at the insults to which we were exposed, and there was a constant feeling of insecurity from the great extent to which we were dependent upon wretches whom we internally despised. When the government took a higher tone, and more principle and greater strictness in the collection of the duties were enforced, we thought ourselves ruined ; but the reverse has been the case. The duties, no doubt, are now excessively burdensome from their amount; but that is their least evil. If it was possible to collect them from every trader with perfect equality, our independence would be complete, and our competition would be confined to superiority in morality and skill. Matters are much nearer this point now than they were fifty years ago ; but still they would admit of considerable improvement.' The same individual mentioned, that, in his youth, now seventy years ago, the civil liberty of the people of Scotland was held by a weak tenure. He knew instances of soldiers being sent, in times of war, to the farm-houses, to carry off, by force, young men for the army ; and as this was against the law, they were accused of some imaginary offence, such as a trespass, or an assault, which was proved by false witnesses, and the magistrate, perfectly aware of the farce, and its object, threatened the victim with transportation to the colonies, as a felon, if he would not enlist; which he, of course, unprotected and overwhelmed by power and injustice, was compelled to consent to.

If the same minute representation were given of other departments of private life, during the time of the greatest immoralities on the part of the government, we would find that this paltering with conscience and character in the national proceedings, tended to keep down the morality of the people, and fostered in them a rapacious and gambling spirit, to which many of the evils that have since overtaken us have owed their origin.

But we may take a more extensive view of the subject of national responsibility.

In the American war England desired to gratify her Acquisitiveness and Self-esteem, in opposition to Benevolence and Justice, at the expense of the transatlantic colonies. This roused the animal resentment of the latter, and the lower faculties of the two nations came into collision; that is to say, they made war on each other; England, to support a dominion in direct hostility to the principles which regulate the moral government of the world, in the expectation of becoming rich and powerful by success in that enterprise; the Americans, to assert the supremacy of the higher sentiments, and to become free and independent. According to the principles which I am now unfolding, the greatest misfortune that could have befallen England would have been success, and the greatest advantage failure in her attempt; and the result is now acknowledged to be in exact accordance with these views. If England had subdued the colonies in the American war, every one must see to what an extent her Self-esteem, Acquisitiveness and Destructiveness would have been let loose upon them; this, in the first place, would have roused their animal faculties, and led them to give her all the annoyance in their power, and the fleets and armies requisite to repress this spirit would have far counterbalanced, in expense, all the profits she could have wrung out of the colonists, by extortion and oppression. In the second place, the very exercise of these animal faculties by herself, in opposition to the moral sentiments, would have rendered her government at home an exact parallel of that of the carter in his own family. The same malevolent principles would have overflowed on her own subjects, the government would have felt uneasy, the people rebellious, discontented, and unhappy, and the moral law would have been amply vindicated by the suffering which would have everywhere abounded. The consequences of her failure have been exactly the reverse. America has sprung up into a great and moral nation, and actually contributes ten times more to the wealth of Britain, standing as she now does, in her natural relation to this country, than she ever could have done, as a discontented and oppressed colony. This advantage is reaped without any loss, anxiety, or expense; it flows from the divine institutions, and both nations profit by and rejoice under it. The moral and intellectual rivalry of America, instead of prolonging the predominance of the propensities in Britain, tends strongly to excite the moral sentiments in her people and government; and every day that we live, we are reaping the benefits of this improvement in wiser institutions, deliverence from endless abuses, and a higher and purer spirit pervading every department of the executive administration of the country. Britain, however, did not escape the penalty of her attempt at the infringement of the moral laws. The pages of her history, during the American war, are dark with suffering and gloom, and at this day we groan under the debt and difficulties then partly incurred.

If the world be constituted on the principles of the supremacy of the moral sentiments and intellect, the method of one nation seeking riches and power, by conquering, devastating, or obstructing the prosperity of other states, must be *essentially futile.* Being in opposition to the moral constitution of creation, it must occasion misery while in progress, and can lead to no result except the impoverishment and mortification of the people who pursue it. The national debt of Britain has been contracted chiefly in wars, originating in commercial jealousy and thirst of conquest ; in short, under the suggestions of Combativeness, Destructiveness, Acquisitiveness, and Self-esteem. Did not our ancestors, therefore, impede their own prosperity and happiness, by engaging in these contests? and have any consequences of them reached us, except the burden of paying nearly thirty millions of taxes annually, as the price of the gratification of their propensities? Would a statesman, who believed in the doctrine of this Essay, have recommended these wars *as essential to national prosperity?* If the twentieth part of the sums had been sent in objects recognised by the moral sentiments, for example, in instituting seminaries of education, penitentiaries, making roads, canals, public granaries, &c. how different would have been the present condition of the country!

After the American, followed the French Revolutionary war. Opinions are at present more divided upon this subject; but my view of it, offered with the greatest deference, is the following. When the French Revolution broke out, the domestic institutions of England were, to a considerable extent, founded and administered on principles in opposition to the supremacy of the sentiments. A clamour was raised by the nation for reform of abuses. If my leading principle is sound, every departure from the moral law in nations, as well as in individuals, carries its punishment with it from the first hour of its commencement, till its final cessation ; and if Britain's institutions were then, to any extent, corrupt and defective, she could not too speedily have abandoned them, and adopted purer and loftier arrangements. Her government, however, clung to the suggestions of the propensities, and resisted every innovation. To divert the national mind from causing a revolution at home, they embarked in a war abroad; and, for a period of twenty-three years, let loose the propensities on France with headlong fury, and a fearful perseverance. France, no doubt, threatened the different nations of Europe with the most violent interference with their governments; a menace wholly unjustifiable, and that called for resistance. But the rulers of that country were preparing their own destruction, in exact proportion to their departures from the moral law; and a statesman, who knew and had confidence in the constitution of the world, as now explained, could have listened to the storm in complete composure, prepared to repel actual aggression, and left the exploding of French infatuation to the Ruler of the Universe, in unhesitating reliance on the efficacy of his laws. But England preferred a war of aggression. If this conduct was in accordance with the sentiments, we should now, like America, be reaping the reward of our obedience to the moral law, and plenty and rejoicing should flow down our streets like a stream. But mark the contrast. This island exhibits the spectacle of millions of men, toiled to the extremity of human endurance, for a pittance scarcely sufficient to sustain life; weavers labouring for fourteen or sixteen hours a day for eightpence, and frequently unable to procure work, even on these terms; other artisans exhausted almost to death by laborious drudgery, who, if better recompensed, seek compensensation and enjoyment in the grossest sensual debauchery, drunkenness, and gluttony; master-traders and manufacturers anxiously labouring for wealth, now gay in the fond hope that all their expectations will be realized, then sunk in deep despair by the breath of ruin having passed over them; land-holders and tenants now reaping unmeasured returns from their properties, then pining in penury, amidst an overflow of every species of produce; the government cramped by an overwhelming debt and the prevalence of ignorance and selfishness on every side, so that it is impossible for it to follow with a bold step the most obvious dictates of reason and justice, owing to the countless prejudices and imaginary interests which every where obstruct the path of improvement. This resembles much more punishment for transgression, than reward for obedience to the divine institutions.

If every man in Britain will turn his attention inwards, and reckon the pangs of disappointment which he has felt at the subversion of his own most darling schemes, by unexpected turns of public events, or the deep inroads on his happiness which such calamities, overtaking his dearest relations and friends, have occasioned to him; the numberless little enjoyments in domestic life, which he is forced to deny himself, by the taxation with which they are loaded; the obstructions to the fair exercise of his industry and talents presented by stamps, licences, excise laws, custom-house duties *et hoc genus omne;* he will discover the extent of responsibility attached by the Creator to national transgressions. From my own observation, I would say, that the miseries inflicted upon individuals and families, by fiscal prosecutions, founded on excise laws, stamp laws, post-office laws, &c. all originating in the necessity of providing for the national debt, are equal to those arising from some of the most extensive natural calamities. It is true, that few persons are prosecuted without having offended; but the evil consists in presenting men with enormous temptations to infringe mere financial regulations not always in accordance with natural morality, and then inflicting ruinous penalties for transgression. Men have hitherto expected the punishment of their offences in the thunderbolt, or the yawning earthquake; and believed, that because the sea did not swallow them up, or the mountain fall upon them and crush them to atoms, Heaven was taking no cognizance of their sins; while, in point of fact, an omnipotent, an all-just, and an all-wise God, had arranged before they erred, an ample retribution in the very consequences of their transgressions. It is by looking to the *principles* in the mind, from which transgressions flow, and attending to their whole operations and results, that we discover the real theory of the divine government. When men shall be instructed in the laws of creation, they will discriminate more accurately than heretofore between natural and factitious evils, and become less tolerant of the latter.

The Spaniards, under the influence of Acquisitiveness, Self-esteem, Love of Approbation, and a blind Veneration, conquered South America, inflicted upon its wretched inhabitants the most atrocious cruelties, and continued to weigh, for three hundred years, like a moral incubus, upon that quarter of the globe. The responsibility now shows itself. By the laws of the Creator, nations require to obey the moral law to be happy; that is, to cultivate the arts of peace, to be industrious, upright, intelligent, pious and humane. The reward of such conduct is individual happiness, and national greatness and glory. There shall then be none to make them afraid. The Spaniards disobeyed all these laws in the conquest of America, they looked to rapine and foreign gold, and not to industry, for wealth; this fostered avarice and pride in the government, baseness in the nobles, indolence, ignorance, and mental depravity in the people; led them to imagine happiness to consist, not in the exercise of the moral and intellectual powers, but in the gratification of all the inferior feelings to the outrage of the higher. Intellectual cultivation was utterly neglected, the sentiments ran astray into the regions of bigotry and superstition, and the propensities acquired a fearful ascendency. These causes made them the prey of internal discord and foreign invaders; and Spain, at this moment, suffers an awful responsibility.*

---

* Cowper recognises these principles of divine government as to nations, and has embodied them in the following powerful verses.

> The hand that slew till it could slay no more,
> Was glued to the sword-hilt with Indian gore.
> Their prince, as justly seated on his throne
> As vain imperial Philip on his own,
> Tricked out of all his royalty by art,
> That stript him bare, and broke his honest heart,
> Died by the sentence of a shaven priest,
> For scorning what they taught him to detest.
> How dark the veil, that intercepts the blaze
> Of Heaven's mysterious purposes and ways;
> God stood not, though he seemed to stand aloof;
> At this hour the conqueror feels the proof;
> The wreath he won drew down an instant curse,
> The fretting plague is in the public purse,
> The cankered spoil corrodes the pining state,
> Starved by that indolence their minds create.
>
> Oh! could their ancient Incas rise again,
> How would they take up Israel's taunting strain!
> Art thou too fallen, Iberia? Do we see
> The robber and the murderer weak as we?
> Thou that hast wasted Earth, and dared despise
> Alike the wrath and mercy of the skies,
> Thy pomp is in the grave, thy glory laid
> Low in the pits thine avarice has made.
> We come with joy from our eternal rest,
> To see th' oppressor in his turn oppressed.
> Art thou the god, the thunder of whose hand
> Rolled over all our desolated land,
> Shook principalities and kingdoms down,
> And made the mountains tremble at his frown?
> The sword shall light upon thy boasted powers,
> And waste them, as the sword has wasted ours.
> 'Tis thus Omnipotence his law fulfils,
> And Vengeance executes what Justice wills.
>
> *Cowper's Poems.—Charity*, p. 156.

In surveying the present aspect of Europe, we perceive astonishing improvements achieved in physical science. How much is implied in the mere names of the steam-engine, power-looms, rail-roads, steam-boats, canals, and gas-lights; and yet of how much misery are several of these inventions at present the direct sources, in consequence of being almost exclusively dedicated to the gratification of the propensities. The leading purpose to which the steam-engine in almost all its forms of application is devoted, is the accumulation of wealth, or the gratification of Acquisitiveness and Self-esteem; and few have proposed, by its means, to lessen the hours of toil to the lower orders of society, so as to afford them opportunity and leisure for the cultivation of their moral and intellectual faculties, and thereby to enable them to render a more perfect obedience to the Creator's institutions. Physical has far outstripped moral science; and, it appears to me, that, unless the lights of Phrenology open the eyes of mankind to the real constitution of the world, and at length induce them to modify their conduct, in harmony with the laws of the Creator, their future physical discoveries will tend only to deepen their wretchedness. Intellect, acting as the ministering servant of the propensities, will lead them only further astray. The science of man's whole nature, animal, moral, and intellectual, was never more required to guide him than at present, when he seems to wield a giant's power, yet in the application of it to display the ignorant selfishness, wilfulness, and absurdity of an overgrown child. History has not yielded, and cannot yield, half her fruits, until mankind shall be possessed of a true theory of their own nature.

SECTION IV.

MORAL ADVANTAGES OF PUNISHMENT.

After the intellect and moral sentiments have been brought to recognise the principles of the Divine administration, so much wisdom, benevolence, and justice, are discernible in the natural laws, that our whole nature is meliorated in undergoing the punishments annexed to them. Punishment endured by one individual also serves to warn others against transgression. These facts afford another proof that a grand object of the arrangement of creation is the improvement of the moral and intellectual nature of man. So strikingly conspicuous, indeed, is the meliorating influence of suffering, that many persons have supposed this to be the primary object for which it is sent ; a notion which, with great deference, appears to me to be unfounded in principle, and dangerous in practice. If evils and misfortunes are mere mercies of providence, it follows that a headache consequent on a debauch, is not intended to prevent a repetition of drunkenness, so much as to prepare the debauchee for ' the invisible world ;' and that shipwreck in a crazy vessel is not designed to render the merchant more cautious, but to lead him to heaven.

It is however undeniable, that in innumerable instances pain and sorrow are the direct consequences of our own misconduct ; at the same time it is obviously benevolent in the Deity to render it beneficial directly as a warning against future transgression, and indirectly as a means of purifying the mind ; nevertheless, if we shall imagine that in some instances it is dispensed as a direct punishment for particular transgressions, and in others, only on account of sin in general, and with the view of meliorating the spirit of the sufferer, we shall ascribe inconsistency to the Creator, and expose ourselves to the danger of attributing our own afflictions to his favour, and those of others, to his wrath; thus fostering in our minds self-conceit and uncharitableness. Individuals who entertain the belief that bad health, worldly ruin, and sinister accidents, befalling them, are not punishments for infringement of the laws of nature, but particular manifestations of the love of the Creator towards themselves, make slight inquiry into the natural causes of their miseries, and bestow few efforts to remove them. In consequence, the chastisements endured by them, neither correct their own conduct, nor deter others from committing similar transgressions. Some religious sects, who espouse these notions, literally act upon them, and refuse to inoculate with the cow-pox to escape contagion, or take other means of avoiding natural calamities. Regarding these as dispensations of Providence, sent to prepare them for a future world, they conceive that the more of them the better. Further; these ideas, besides being repugnant to the common sense of mankind, are at variance with the principle that the world is arranged so as to favour virtue and discountenance vice; because favouring virtue means obviously that the favoured virtuous will positively enjoy more happiness, and, negatively, suffer fewer misfortunes than the vicious. The view, then, now advocated, appears less exceptionable, viz. that punishment serves a double purpose, directly to warn us against transgression; and indirectly, when rightly apprehended, to subdue our lower propensities, and purify and vivify our moral and intellectual powers.

Bishop BUTLER coincides in this interpretation of natural calamities. 'Now,' says he, 'in the present state, all which we enjoy, *and* A GREAT PART OF WHAT WE SUFFER, *is put in our power.** For *pleasure and pain are the consequences of our actions;* and we are endued by the Autor of our nature with capacities of foreseeing these con-

---

* These words are printed in Italics in the original.

sequences.' 'I know not that we have any one kind or degree of enjoyment, but by the means of our own actions. And, *by prudence and care,* we may, for the most part, pass our days in tolerable ease and quiet ; or, on the contrary, we may, *by rashness, ungoverned passion, wilfulness,* or *even by negligence,* make ourselves *as miserable as ever we please.* And many do please to make themselves extremely miserable ; *i. e.* they do what they knew beforehand will render them so. They follow those ways, the fruit of which they knew, by instruction, example, experience, will be disgrace, and poverty, and sickness, and untimely death. This every one observes to be the general course of things ; though it is to be allowed, we cannot find by experience, that *all* our sufferings are owing to our own follies.'—*Analogy*, p. 40. In accordance with this last remark, I have treated of *hereditary* diseases ; and evils resulting from convulsions of physical nature may be added to the same class.

It has been objected that physical punishments, such as the breaking of an arm by a fall, are often so disproportionally severe, that the Creator must have had some other and more important object in view in appointing them, than to serve as mere motives to physical observance ; and that that object must be to influence the mind of the sufferer, and to draw his attention to concerns of higher import.

In answer, I remark, that the human body is liable to destruction by severe injuries ; and that the degree of suffering, in general, bears a just proportion to the danger connected with the transgression. Thus, a slight surfeit is attended only with headache or general uneasiness, because it does not endanger life ; a fall on any muscular part of the body is followed either with no pain, or only a slight indisposition, for the reason that it is not seriously injurious to life ; but when a leg or arm is broken, the pain is intensely severe, because the bones of these limbs stand high in the scale of utility to man. The human body is so framed that it may fall nine times, and suffer little damage, but the tenth time a limb may be broken, which will entail a painful chastisement. By this arrangement the mind is kept alive to danger to such an extent, as to ensure general safety, while at the same time it is not overwhelmed with terror by punishments too severe and too frequently repeated. In particular states of the body, a slight wound may be followed by inflammation and death; but these are not the results simply of the wound, but the consequences of a previous derangement of health, occasioned by departures from the organic laws.

On the whole, therefore, no adequate reason appears for regarding the consequences of physical accidents in any other light than as direct punishments for infringement of the natural laws, and indirectly as a means of accomplishing moral and religious improvement.

CHAPTER IV.

ON THE COMBINED OPERATION OF THE NATURAL LAWS.

Having now unfolded several of the natural laws, and their effects, and having also attempted to show that each is inflexible and independent in itself, and requires absolute obedience, so that a man who shall neglect the physical law will suffer the physical punishment, although he may be very attentive to the moral law; that one who infringes the organic law will suffer organic punishment, although he may obey the physical law; and that a person who violates the moral law will suffer the moral punishment, although he should observe the other two; I proceed to show the mutual relationship between these laws, and to adduce some instances of their joint operation.

The great fires in Edinburgh, in November, 1824, when the Parliament Square and a part of the High Street were consumed, will serve as one example. That calamity may be viewed in the following light:—The Creator constituted the countries of England and Scotland, and the English and Scottish nations, with such qualities and relationships, that the individuals of both kingdoms would be most happy in acting towards each other, and pursuing their separate vocations, under the supremacy of the moral sentiments. We have lived to see this practised, and to reap the rewards of it. But the ancestors of the two nations did not believe in this constitution of the world, and they preferred acting on the principles of the propensities; that is to say, they waged furious wars, and committed wasting devastations, on each other's properties and lives. This was clearly a violent infringement of the moral law; and it is obvious from history that the two nations were equally ferocious, and delighted reciprocally in each other's calamities. One effect of it was to render personal safety an object of paramount importance. The hill on which the Old Town of Edinburgh is built, was naturally surrounded by marshes, and presented a perpendicular front, to the west, capable of being crowned with a castle. It was appropriated with avidity, and the metropolis of Scotland founded there, obviously and undeniably under the inspiration purely of the animal faculties. It was fenced round, and ramparts built to exclude the fierce warriors who then inhabited the south of the Tweed, and also to protect the inhabitants from the feudal banditti who infested their own soil. The space within the walls, however, was limited and narrow; the attractions to the spot were numerous, and to make the most of it, our ancestors erected the enormous masses of high, confused, and crowded buildings which now compose the High Street of this city, and the wynds, or alleys, on its two sides. These abodes, moreover, were constructed, to a great extent, of timber, for not only the joists and floors, but the partitions between the rooms, were of massive wood. Our ancestors did all this in the perfect knowledge of the physical law, that wood ignited by fire is not only consumed itself, but envelopes in inevitable destruction every combustible object within its influence. Further ; their successors, even when the necessity had ceased, persevered in the original error, and in the perfect knowledge that every year added to the age of such fabrics increased their liability to burn, they allowed them to be occupied not only as shops filled with paper, spirits, and other highly combustible materials, but introduced gaslights, and let off the upper floors for brothels, introducing thereby into the heart of this magazine of conflagration, the most reckless and immoral of mankind. The consummation was the tremendous fires of November, 1824, the one originating in a whiskey-cellar, and the other in a garret brothel, which consumed the whole Parliament Square and a part of the High Street, destroying property to the extent of many thousands of pounds, and spreading misery and ruin over a considerable portion of the population of Edinburgh. Wonder, consternation, and awe were forcibly excited at the vastness of this calamity ; and in the sermons that were preached, and the dissertations that were written upon it, much was said of the inscrutable ways of Providence, that sent such visitations upon the poople, enveloping the innocent and the guilty in one common sentence of destruction.

According to the exposition of the ways of Providence which I have ventured to give, there was nothing wonderful, nothing vengeful, nothing arbitrary, in the whole occurrence. The surprising thing was, that it did not take place generations before. The necessity for these fabrics originated in gross violation of the moral law; they were constructed in high contempt of the physical law ; and, latterly, the moral law was set at defiance, by placing in them inhabitants abandoned to the worst habits of recklessness and intoxication. The Creator had bestowed on men faculties to perceive all this, and to avoid it, whenever they chose to exert them; and the destruction that ensued was the punishment of following the propensities, in preference to the dictates of intellect and morality. The object of the destruction, as a natural event, was to lead men to avoid repetition of the offences: but the principles of the divine government are not yet comprehended; Acquisitiveness whispers that more money may be made of houses consisting of five or six floors, under one roof, than of only two; and erections, the very counterparts of the former, are now rearing their heads on the spot where the others stood, and, sooner or later, they also will be overtaken by the natural laws, which never slumber or sleep.

The true method of arriving at a sound view of calamities of every kind, is to direct our attention, in the first instance, to the law of nature, from the operation of which they have originated; then to find out the uses and advantages of that law when observed; and to discover whether the evils under consideration have arisen from violation of it. In the present instance, we ought never to lose sight of the fact, that the houses in question stood erect, and the furniture in safety, by the very same law of gravitation which made them topple to the foundation when it was infringed; that mankind enjoy all the benefits which result from the combustibility of timber as fuel, by the very same law which renders it a devouring element, when unduly ignited; that, by the same moral law, which, when infringed, leads to the necessity of ramparts, fortifications, crowded lanes, and extravagantly high houses, we enjoy, now that we observe it better, that security of property and life which distinguishes modern Scotland from ancient Caladonia.

This instance affords a striking illustration of the manner in which the physical and organic laws are constituted in harmony with, and in subserviency to, the moral law. We see clearly that the leading cause of the construction of such erections as the houses of the Old Town of Edinburgh (with the deprivation of free air, and liability to combustion that attend them), arose from the excessive predominance of Combativeness, Destructiveness, Self-esteem, and Acquisitiveness, in our ancestors; and although the ancient personages who erected these monuments of animal supremacy, had no conception that, in doing so, they were laying the foundations of a severe punishment on themselves and their posterity; yet, when we compare the comforts and advantages that would have accompanied dwellings constructed under the inspiration of Benevolence, Ideality, and enlightened Intellect, with the contaminating, debasing, and dangerous effects of their workmanship, we perceive most clearly that they actually were the instruments of chastising their own transgressions, and of transmitting that chastisement to their posterity, so long as the animal supremacy shall be prolonged. Another example may be given.

Men, uniting under one leader, may, in virtue of the social law, acquire prodigious advantages to themselves, which singly they could not obtain; and I stated, that the condition under which the benefits of that law were permitted, was, that the leader should know and obey the natural laws that were conducive to success; if he neglected these, then the same principle which gave the social body the benefit of his observing them, involved them in the punishment of his infringement; and that this was just, because, under the natural law, the leader must necessarily be chosen by the social body, and they were responsible for not attending to his natural qualities. Some illustrations of the consequences of neglect of this law may be stated, in which the mixed operation of the physical and moral laws will appear.

During the French war, a squadron of English men-of-war was sent to the Baltic with military stores, and, in returning home up Channel, they were beset, for two or three days, by a thick fog. It was about the middle of December, and no correct information was possessed of their exact situation. Some of the commanders proposed lying-to all night, and proceeding only during day, to avoid running ashore unawares. The commodore was exceedingly attached to his wife and family, and stated his determination to pass Christmas with them in England, if possible, and ordered the ships to sail straight on their voyage. The very same night they all struck on a sand-bank off the coast of Holland; two ships of the line were dashed to pieces, and every soul on board perished. The third ship drew less water, was forced over the bank by the waves, was stranded on the beach, the crew saved, but led to a captivity of many years' duration. Now, these vessels were destroyed under the physical law; but this calamity owed its origin to the predominance of the animal over the moral and intellectual faculties in the commodore. The gratification which he sought to obtain was individual and selfish; and, if his Benevolence, Veneration, Conscientiousness, and Intellect, had been as alert and carried as forcibly home to his mind the operation of the physical laws, and the welfare of the men under his charge; nay, if these faculties had been sufficiently alive to see the danger to which he exposed his own life, and the happiness of his own wife and children,—he never could have followed the precipitate course which consigned himself, and so many brave men, to a watery grave, within a few hours after his resolution was formed.

Very lately the Ogle Castle East Indiaman was offered a pilot coming up Channel, but the captain refused assistance, professing his own skill to be sufficient. In a few hours the ship ran aground on a sand-bank, and every human being perished in the waves. This also arose from the physical law, but the unfavourable operation of it sprung from Self-esteem, pretending to knowledge which the intellect did not possess ; and, as it is only by the latter that obedience can be yielded to the physical laws, the destruction of the ship was indirectly the consequence of infringement of the moral and intellectual laws.

An old sailor, whom I lately met on the Queens-ferry passage, told me, that he had been nearly fifty years at sea, and once was in a fifty gun ship in the West Indies. The captain, he said, was a ' fine man ;' he knew the climate, and foresaw a hurricane coming, by its natural signs ; and, on one occasion, in particular, he struck the top-masts, lowered the yards, lashed the guns, made each man supply himself with food for thirty-six hours, and scarcely was this done when the hurricane came ; the ship lay for four hours on her beam-ends in the water ; but all was prepared ; the men were kept in vigour during the storm and fit for every exertion ; the ship at last righted, suffered little damage, and proceeded on her voyage. The fleet which she convoyed was dispersed, and a great number of the ships foundered. Here we see the supremacy of the moral and intellectual faculties, and discover to what a surprising extent they present a guarantee, even against the fury of the physical elements in their highest state of agitation.

One of the most instructive illustrations of the connexion between the different natural laws is presented in Captain Lyon's brief narrative of an unsuccessful attempt to reach Repulse Bay, in his Majesty's ship Griper, in the year 1824.

Captain Lyon mentions, that he sailed in the Griper on 13th June, 1824, in company with his Majesty's surveying vessel Snap, as a store-tender. The Griper was 180 tons burden, and ' drew 16 feet 1 inch abaft, and 15 feet 10 inches forward.'—p. 2. On the 26th, he, ' was sorry to observe that the Griper, from her great depth and sharpness forward, pitched very deeply.'—p. 3. ' She sailed so ill, that 'in a stiff breeze and with studding-sails set, he was unable to get above four knots an hour out of her, and she was twice whirled round in an eddy in the Pentland Frith, from which she could not escape.'—p. 6. On the 3d July, 'being now fairly at sea, I caused the Snap to take us in tow, which I had declined doing as we passed up the east coast of England, although our little companion had much difficulty in keeping under sufficiently low sail for us, and by noon we had passed the Stack Back.' 'The Snap was of the greatest assistance, the Griper frequently towing at the rate of five knots, in cases where she would not have gone three.'—p. 10. 'On the forenoon of the 16th, the Snap came and took us in tow; but at noon on the 17th, strong breezes and a heavy swell obliged us again to cast off. We scudded while able, but our depth on the water caused us to ship so many heavy seas, that I most reluctantly brought to under storm stay-sails. This was rendered exceedingly mortifying, by observing that our companion was perfectly dry, and not affected by the sea.'—p. 13. 'When our stores were all on board, we found our narrow decks completely crowded by them. The gangways, forecastle, and abaft the mizen-mast, were filled with casks, hawsers, whale-lines, and stream-cables, while on our straitened lower decks we were obliged to place casks and other stores, in every part but that allotted to the ship's company's mess-tables; and even my cabin had a quantity of things stowed away in it.'—p. 21. 'It may be proper to mention, that the *Fury* and *Hecla*, which were enabled to stow *three* years provisions, were each exactly *double* the size of the Griper, and the Griper carried two years' and a half's provisions.'—pp. 22, 23.

Arrived in the Polar Seas, they were visited by a storm, of which Captain Lyon gives the following description:—
'We soon, however, came to fifteen fathoms, and I kept right away, but had then only ten; when, being unable to see far around us, and observing, from the whiteness of the

water, that we were on a bank, I rounded to at 7 A. M., and tried to bring up with the starboard anchor, and seventy fathoms chain, but the stiff breeze and heavy sea caused this to part in half an hour, and we again made sail to the north east-ward; but finding we came suddenly to seven fathoms, and that the ship could not possibly work out again, as she would not face the sea, or keep steerage-way on her, I most reluctantly brought her up with three bowers and a stream in succession, yet not before we had shoaled to five and a half. This was between 8 and 9 A. M., the ship pitching bows under, and a tremendous sea running. At noon the starboard-bower anchor parted, but the others held.

'As there was every reason to fear the falling of the tide, which we knew to be from twelve to fifteen feet on this coast, and in that case the total destruction of the ship, I caused the longboat to be hoisted out, and with the four smaller ones to be stored to a certain extent, with arms and provisions. The officers drew lots for their respective boats, and the ship's company were stationed to them. The longboat having been filled full of stores, which could not be put below, it became requisite to throw them overboard, *as there was no room for them on our very small and crowded decks, over which heavy seas were constantly sweeping.* In making these preparations for taking to the boats, it was evident to all, that the longboat was the only one that had the slightest chance of living under the lee of the ship, should she be wrecked, but every officer and man drew his lot with the greatest composure, though two of our boats would have swamped the instant they were lowered. Yet, such was the noble feeling of those around me, that it was evident, that, had I ordered the boats in question to be manned, their crews would have entered them without a murmur. In the afternoon, on the weather clearing a little, we discovered a low beach all around astern of us, on which the surf was running to an awful height, and it appeared evident that no human powers could save us. At 3 p. m. the tide had fallen, twentytwo feet, *(only six feet more than we drew,)* and the ship, having been lifted up by a tremendous sea, struck with great violence the length of her keel. This we naturally conceived was the forerunner of her total wreck, and we stood in readiness to take the boats, and endeavour to hang under her lee. She continued to strike with sufficient force to have burst any less fortified vessel, at intervals of a few minutes, whenever an unusual heavy sea passed us. And, as the water was so shallow, these might almost be called breakers rather than waves, for each in passing burst with great force over our gangways, and as every sea 'topped,' our decks were continually, and frequently, deeply flooded. All hands took a little refreshment, for some had scarcely been below for twentyfour hours, and I had not been in bed for three nights. Although few, or none of us, had any idea that we should survive the gale, we did not think that our comforts should be entirely neglected, and an order was therefore given to the men to put on their best and warmest clothing, to enable them to support life as long as possible. Every man therefore, brought his bag on deck, and dressed himself; and in the fine athletic forms which stood before me, I did not see one muscle quiver, nor the slightest sign of alarm. The officers each secured some useful instrument about them, for the purpose of observation, although it was acknowledged by all that not the slightest hope remained. And now that every thing in our power had been done, I called all hands aft, and to a merciful God offered prayers for our preservation. I thanked every one for their excellent conduct, and cautioned them, as we should, in all probability, soon appear before our Maker, to enter his presence as men resigned to their fate. We then all sat down in groups, and, sheltered from the wash of the sea, by whatever we could find, many of us endeavoured to obtain a little sleep. Never, perhaps, was witnessed a finer scene than on the deck of my little ship, when all the hope of life had left us. Noble as the character of the British sailor is always allowed to be in cases of danger; yet I did not believe it to be possible, that, among forty-one persons, not one repining word should have been uttered. The officers sat about, wherever they could find a shelter from the sea, and the men lay down conversing with each other with the most perfect calmness. Each was at peace with his neighbour and all the world, and I am firmly persuaded that the resignation which was then shown to the will of the almighty, was the means of obtaining his mercy. At about 6 p. m., the rudder, which had already received some very heavy blows, rose and broke up the after-lockers, and this was the last severe shock that the ship received. We found by the well that she made no water, and by dark she struck no more. God was merciful to us, and the tide almost miraculously fell no lower. At dark heavy rain fell, but was borne in patience, for it beat down the gale, and brought with it a light air from the northward. At nine p. m,. the water had deepened to five fathoms. The ship kept off the ground all night, and our exhausted crew obtained some broken rest.'—p. 76.

In humble gratitude for his deliverance, he called the place ' The Bay of God's mercy,' and ' offered up thanks and praises to God, for the mercy he had shown to us.'

On 12th September, they had another gale of wind, with cutting showers of sleet, and a heavy sea. *' At such a time as this,'* says Captain Lyon, *' we had fresh cause to deplore the extreme dulness of the Griper's sailing, for though almost any other vessel would have worked off this lea-shore, we made little or no progress on a wind, but remained actually pitching, forecastle under, with scarcely steerage-way,* to preserve which I was ultimately obliged to keep her nearly two points off the wind.'—p. 98.

Another storm overtook them, which is described as follows:—' Never shall I forget the dreariness of this most anxious night. Our ship pitched at such a rate that it was not possible to stand, even below; while on deck we were unable to move, without holding by ropes, which were stretched from side to side. The drift snow flew in such sharp heavy flakes, that we could not look to windward, and it froze on deck to above a foot in depth. The sea made incessant breaches quite fore and aft the ship, and the temporary warmth it gave while it washed over us, was most painfully checked, by its almost immediately freezing on our clothes. To these discomforts were added, the horrible uncertainty as to whether the cables would hold until daylight, and the conviction also, that if they failed us, we should instantly be dashed to pieces; the wind blowing directly to the quarter in which we knew the shore must lie. Again, should they continue to hold us, we feared, by the ship's complaining so much forward, that the bitts would be torn up, or that she would settle down at her anchors, overpowered by some of the tremendous seas which burst over her. At dawn on the 13th, thirty minutes after four A. M., we found that the best bower cable had parted; and, as the gale now blew with terrific violence from the north, there was little reason to expect that the other anchors would hold long; or, if they did, we *pitched so deeply, and lifted so great a body of water each time, that it was feared the windlass and forecastle would be torn up, or she must go down at her anchors;* although the ports were knocked out, and a considerable portion of the bulwark cut away, she could scarcely discharge one sea before shipping another, and the decks were frequently flooded to an alarming depth.

' At six A. M., all further doubts on this particular account were at an end; for, having received two overwhelming seas, both the other cables went at the same moment, and we were left helpless, without anchors, or any means of saving ourselves, should the shore, as we had every reason to expect, be close astern. And here, again, I had the happiness of witnessing the same general tranquillity as was shown on the 1st of September. There was no outcry that the cables were gone; but my friend Mr. Manico, with Mr. Carr the gunner, came aft as soon as they recovered their legs, and, in the lowest whisper, informed me that the cables had all parted. The ship, in trending to the wind, lay quite down on her broadside, and as it then became evident that nothing held her, and that she was quite helpless, each man instinctively took his station; while the seamen at the leads, having secured themselves as well as was in their power, repeated their soundings, on which our preservation depended, with as much composure as if we had been entering a friendly port. Here, again, that Almighty power, which had before so mercifully preserved us, granted us his protection.'—p. 100.

Nothing can be more interesting and moving than this narrative; it displays a great predominance of the moral sentiments and intellect, but sadly unenlightened as to the natural laws. I quoted, in Captain LYON's own words, his description of the Griper, loaded to such excess that she drew sixteen feet water; that she was incapable of sailing; that she was whirled round in an eddy in the Pentland Frith; that seas broke over her that did not wet the deck of the little Snap, not half her size. Captain LYON knew all this; and also the roughness of the climate to which he was steering; and, with these outrages of the physical law staring him in the face, he proceeded on his voyage, without addressing, so far as we perceive, one remonstrance to the Lords of the Admiralty on the subject of this infringement of every principle of common prudence. My opinion is, that Captain LYON was not blind to the errors committed in his equipment, or to their probable consequences; but that his powerful sentiment of Veneration, combined with Cautiousness and Love of Approbation, (misdirected in this instance,) deprived him of courage to complain to the Admiralty, through fear of giving offence: or that, if he did complain, they have prevented him from stating the fact in his narrative. To the tempestuous north he sailed; and his greatest dangers were clearly referable to the very infringements of the physical laws which he describes. When the tide ebbed, his ship reached to within six feet of the bottom, and, in the hollow of every wave, struck with great violence: but she was loaded at least four feet too deeply, by his own account; so that, if he had done his own duty, she would have had four feet of additional water, or, ten feet in all, between her and the bottom, even in the hollow of the wave,—a matter of the very last importance, in such a critical condition. Indeed, with four feet more water, she would not have struck. Besides, if less loaded, she would have struck less violently. Again, when pressed upon a lea shore, her incapability of sailing was a most obvious cause of danger: in short, if Providence is to be regarded as the cause of these calamities, there is no impropriety which man can commit, which may not, on the same principles, be charged against the Creator.

But the moral law again shines forth in delightful splendour, in the conduct of Captain Lyon and his crew, when in the most forlorn condition. Piety, resignation, and manly resolution, then animated them to the noblest efforts. On the principle, that the power of accommodating the conduct to the natural laws, depends on the activity of the sentiments and intellect, and that the more numerous the faculties that are excited, the greater is the energy communicated to the whole system, I would say, that, while Captain Lyon's sufferings were, in a great degree, brought on by his infringements of the physical laws, his escape was, in a great measure, promoted by his obedience to the moral law; and that Providence, in the whole occurrence, proceeded on the broad and general principle, which sends advantage uniformly as the reward of obedience, and evil as the punishment of infringement, of every particular law of creation.

That storms and tempests have been instituted for some benevolent end, may, perhaps, be acknowledged, when their causes and effects are fully known, which at present is not the case. But, even amidst all our ignorance of these, it is surprising how small a portion of evil they would occasion, if men obeyed the laws which are actually ascertained. How many ships perish from being sent to sea in an old worn out condition, and ill equipped, through mere Acquisitiveness; and how many more, from captains and crews being chosen who are greatly deficient in knowledge, intelligence, and morality, in consequence of which they infringe the physical laws. We ought to look to all these matters, before complaining of storms as natural institutions.

The last example of the mixed operation of the natural laws which I shall notice, is that which followed from the mercantile distresses of 1825-6. I have traced the origin of that visitation to excessive activity of Acquisitiveness, and a general ascendency of the animal and selfish faculties over the moral and intellectual powers. The punishments of these offences were manifold. The excesses infringed the moral law, and the chastisement for this was deprivation of the tranquil, steady enjoyment that flows only from the sentiments, with severe suffering in the ruin of fortune and blasting of hope. These disappointments produced mental anguish and depression; which occasioned unhealthy action in the brain. The action of the brain being disturbed, a morbid nervous influence was transmitted to the whole corporeal system; bodily disease was superadded to mental sorrow, and, in some instances, the unhappy sufferers committed suicide to escape from these aggravated evils. Under the organic law, the children produced in this period of mental depression, bodily distress, and organic derangement, will inherit weak bodies, with feeble and irritable minds, a hereditary chastisement of their father's transgressions.

In the instances now given, we discover the various laws acting in perfect harmony, and in subordination to the moral and intellectual. If our ancestors had not forsaken the supremacy of the moral sentiments, such fabrics as the houses in the Old Town of Edinburgh never would have been built; and if the modern proprietors had returned to that law, and kept profligate and drunken inhabitants out of them, the conflagration might still have been avoided. In the case of the ships, we saw, that wherever intellect and sentiment had been relaxed, and animal motives permitted to assume the supremacy, evil had speedily followed ; and that where the higher powers were called forth, safety had been obtained. And, finally, in the case of the merchants and manufacturers, we traced their calamities directly to placing Acquisitiveness and Ambition above Intellect and Sentiment.

Formidable and appalling, then, as these punishments are, yet, when we attend to the laws under which they occur, and perceive that the object and legitimate operation of every one of them, when observed, is to produce happiness to man ; and that the punishments have the sole object in view of forcing him back to this enjoyment, we cannot, under the supremacy of the sentiments and intellect, fail to bow in humility before them, and at once wise, just, and beneficent.

CONCLUSION.

The question has frequently been asked, What is the practical use of Phrenology, even supposing it to be true? A few observations will enable us to answer this inquiry; and at the same time, to present a brief summary of the doctrine of the preceding Essay.

Prior to the age of Galileo, the earth and sun presented to the eye phenomena exactly similar to those which they now exhibit; but their motions appeared in a very different light to the understanding.

Before the age of Newton, the revolutions of the planets were known as matter of fact; but the understanding was ignorant of the principle of their motions.

Previous to the dawn of modern chemistry, many of the qualities of physical substances were ascertained by observation, but their ultimate principles and relations were not understood.

Knowledge may be rendered beneficial in two ways,—either by rendering the substance discovered directly subservient to human enjoyment; or, where this is impossible, by modifying human conduct in harmony with its qualities. While knowledge of any department of nature remains imperfect and empirical, the unknown qualities of the objects belonging to it may render our efforts either to apply or to accord with those which are known, altogether abortive. Hence it is only after ultimate principles have been discovered, their relations ascertained, and this knowledge has been systematised, that science can attain its full character of utility. The merits of Galileo and Newton consist in having rendered this service to astronomy.

CONCLUSION.

Before the appearance of Drs. GALL and SPURZHEIM, mankind were practically acquainted with the feelings and intellectual operations of their own minds; and anatomists knew the appearances of the brain: But the science of Mind was very much in the same state as that of the heavenly bodies prior to GALILEO and NEWTON. This remark is borne out by the following considerations:

First. No unanimity prevailed among philosophers concerning the elementary feelings and intellectual powers of man. Individuals, deficient in Conscientiousness, for instance, denied that the sentiment of justice was a primitive mental quality of mind. Others, deficient in Veneration, asserted that man was not naturally prone to worship, and ascribed religion to the invention of priests.

Secondly. The extent to which the primitive faculties differ in relative strength, was matter of dispute, or of vague conjecture; and there was no agreement whether many actual attainments were the gifts of nature, or the results of mere cultivation.

Thirdly. Different modes of the same feeling were often mistaken for different feelings: and modes of action of all the intellectual faculties were mistaken for faculties themselves.

Fourthly. The brain, confessedly the most important organ of the body, and that with which the nerves of the senses, of motion, and of feeling directly communicate, had no ascertained functions. Mankind were ignorant of its uses, and of its influence on the mental faculties. They indeed still dispute that its different parts are the organs of different mental powers, and that the vigour of manifestation bears a proportion, *cæteris paribus*, to the size of the organ.

If, in physics, imperfect and empirical knowledge renders the unknown qualities of bodies liable to frustrate the efforts of man to apply or to accommodate his conduct to their known qualities; and if only a complete and systematic exhibition of ultimate principles, and their relations, can confer on science its full character of utility,—the same doctrine applies with equal or greater force to the philosophy of man. For example,

POLITICS embrace forms of government, and the relations between different states. All government is designed to combine the efforts of individuals, and to regulate their conduct when united. To arrive at the best means of accomplishing this end, systematic knowledge of the nature of man seems highly important. A despotism, for example, may restrain some abuses of the lower propensities, but it assuredly impedes the exercise of reflection, and others of the highest and noblest powers. A form of government can be suited to the nature of man only when it is calculated to permit the legitimate use, and to restrain the abuses, of all his mental feelings and capacities; and how can such a government be devised, while these principles, with their spheres of action, and external relations, are imperfectly ascertained. Again; all relations between different states must also be in accordance with the nature of man, to prove permanently beneficial; and the question recurs, How are these to be framed while that nature is matter of conjecture? NAPOLEON disbelieved in a sentiment of justice as an innate quality of mind; and, in his relations with other states, relied on fear and interest as the grand motives of conduct: but that sentiment existed; and, combined with other faculties which he outraged, prompted Europe to hurl him from his throne. If NAPOLEON had comprehended the principles of human nature, and their relations, as forcibly and clearly as the principles of mathematics, in which he excelled, his understanding would have greatly modified his conduct, and Europe would have escaped prodigious calamities.

LEGISLATION, civil and criminal, is intended to regulate and direct the human faculties in their efforts at gratification; and, to be useful, laws must accord with the constitution of these faculties. But how can salutary laws be enacted, while the subject to be governed, or human nature, is not accurately understood? The inconsistency and intricacy of the laws even in enlightened nations, have afforded themes for the satirist in every age; and how could the case be otherwise? Legislators provided rules for directing the qualities of human nature, which they conceived themselves to know; but either error in their conceptions, or the effects of other qualities unknown or unattended to, defeated their intentions. The law, for example, punishing heresy with burning, was addressed by our ancestors to Cautiousness, Self-Love, and other inferior feelings; but intellect, Veneration, Conscientiousness, and Firmness, were omitted in their estimate of human principles of action; and these set their laws at defiance.

There are many laws still in the statute book, equally at variance with the nature of man.

EDUCATION is intended to enlighten the intellect and moral sentiments, and train them to vigour. But how can this be successfully accomplished, when the faculties and sentiments themselves, the laws to which they are subjected, and their relations to external objects, are unascertained. Accordingly, the theories and practices observed in education are innumerable and contradictory, which could not happen if men knew the constitution of the object which they were training.

MORALS and RELIGION, also, cannot assume a systematic and demonstrable character, until the elementary qualities of mind, and their relations shall be ascertained.

It is presumable that the Deity, in creating the moral powers and the external world, really adapted the one to the other; so that individuals and nations, in pursuing morality, must, in every instance, be promoting their best interests, and, in departing from it, must be sacrificing them to passion, or to illusory notions of advantage. But, until the nature of man, and the relationship between it and the external world, shall be scientifically ascertained, and systematically expounded, it will be impossible to support morality by the powerful demonstration of interest, as here supposed, coinciding with it. The tendency in most men to view expediency as not always coincident with justice, affords a striking proof of the limited knowledge of the constitution of man and the external world still prevalent in society.

The diversities of doctrine in religion also obviously owe their origin to ignorance of the primitive faculties and their relations. The faculties differ in relative strength in different individuals, and each person is most alive to objects and views connected with the powers predominant in himself. Hence, in reading the Scriptures, one is convinced that they establish Calvinism; another, possesssing a different combination of faculties, discovers in them Lutheranism; and a third is satisfied that Socinianism is the only true interpretation. These individuals have, in general, no distinct conception that the views which strike them most forcibly, appear in a different light to minds differently constituted. A correct interpretation of revelation must harmonize with the dictates of the moral sentiments and intellect, holding the animal propensities in subordination. It may legitimately go beyond what they, unaided, could reach; but it cannot contradict them; because this would be setting the revelation of the bible in opposition to the inherent dictates of the faculties constituted by the Creator, which cannot be admitted; as the Deity is too powerful and wise to be inconsistent. But mankind will never be induced to bow to such interpretations, while each takes his individual mind as a standard of human nature in general, and conceives that his own impressions are synonymous with absolute truth. The establishment of the nature of man, therefore, on a scientific basis, and in a systematic form, must aid the cause both of morality and religion.

The PROFESSIONS, PURSUITS, AMUSEMENTS, and HOURS OF EXERTION of individuals, ought also to bear reference to their physical and mental constitution; but hitherto no guiding principle has been possessed to regulate practice in these important particulars,—another evidence that the science of man has been unknown.

But we require only to attend to the scenes daily presenting themselves in society, to obtain irresistible demonstration of the consequences resulting from the want of a true theory of human nature, and its relations. Every preceptor in schools, every professor in colleges, every author, editor, and pamphleteer, every member of Parliament, counsellor and judge, has a set of notions of his own, which in his mind hold the place of a system of the philosophy of man; and although he may not have methodized his ideas, or even acknowledged them to himself as a theory, yet they constitute a standard to him by which he practically judges of all questions in morals, politics, and religion; he advocates whatever views coincide with them, and condemns all that differ from them, with as unhesitating dogmatism as the most pertinacious theorist on earth. Each also despises the notions of his fellows, in so far as they differ from his own. In short, the human faculties too generally operate simply as instincts, exhibiting all the confliction and uncertainty of mere feeling, unenlightened by perception of their own nature and objects. Hence public measures in general, whether relating to education, religion, trade, manufactures, the poor, criminal law, or to any other of the dearest interests of society, instead of being treated as branches of one general system of economy, and adjusted each on scientific principles in harmony with all the rest, are supported or opposed on narrow and empirical grounds, and often call forth displays of ignorance, prejudice, selfishness, intolerance, and bigotry, that greatly obstruct the progress of improvement. Indeed, unanimity, even among sensible and virtuous men, will be impossible, so long as no standard of mental philosophy is admitted to guide individual feelings and perceptions. But the state of things now described could not exist if education embraced a true system of human nature and its relations.

If then, phrenology be true, it will, when matured, supply the deficiencies now pointed out.

But, here, another question naturally presents itself, How are the views now expounded, supposing them to contain some portion of truth, to be rendered practical? In answer I remark, that the institutions and manners of society indicate the state of mind of the influential classes at the time when they prevail. The trial and burning of old women as witches, point out clearly the predominance of Destructiveness and Wonder over Intellect and Benevolence, in those who are guilty of such cruel absurdities. The practices of wager of battle, and ordeal by fire and water, indicate Combativeness, Destructiveness, and Veneration, to have been in great activity in those who permitted them, combined with much intellectual ignorance of the natural constitution of the world. In like manner, the enormous sums willingly expended in war, and the small sums grudgingly paid for public improvements; the intense energy displayed in the pursuit of wealth; and the general apathy evinced in the search after knowledge and virtue, unequivocally proclaim activity of Combativeness, Destructiveness, Acquisitiveness, Self-esteem, and Love of Approbation; with comparatively moderate vivacity of Benevolence and Intellect, in the present generation. Before, therefore, the practices of mankind can be altered, the state of their minds must be changed. No practical error can be greater than that of establishing institutions greatly in advance of the mental condition of the people. The rational method is first to instruct the intellect, then to interest the sentiments, and, last of all, to form arrangements in harmony with, and resting on, these as their basis.

CONCLUSION.

The views developed in the preceding chapters, if founded in nature, may be expected to lead, ultimately, to considerable changes in many of the customs and pursuits of society; but to accomplish this effect, the principles themselves must first be ascertained to be true; then they must be sedulously taught; and when the public mind has been thoroughly prepared, then only ought important practical alterations to be proposed. It appears to me that a long series of years will be necessary to bring even civilized nations into a condition systematically to obey the natural laws.

The preceding chapters may be regarded, in one sense, as an introduction to an Essay on Education. If the views unfolded in them be in general sound, it will follow that education has scarcely yet commenced. If the Creator has bestowed on the body, on the mind, and on external nature, determinate constitutions, and arranged these so as to act on each other, and to produce happiness or misery to man, according to certain definite principles, and if this action goes on invariably, inflexibly, and irresistibly, whether men attend to it or not, it is obvious that the very basis of useful knowledge must consist in an acquaintance with these natural arrangements: and that education will be valuable in the exact degree in which it communicates such information, and trains the faculties to act upon it. Reading, writing, and accounts, which make up the instruction enjoyed by the lower orders, are merely *means of acquiring knowledge*, but do not *constitute* it. Greek, Latin, and mathematics, which are added in the education of the middle classes, are still only *means* of obtaining information; so that, with the exception of the few who pursue physical science, society dedicates very little attention to the study of the natural laws. In following out the views now discussed, therefore, each individual, according as he becomes acquainted with the natural laws, ought to obey them, and to communicate his experience of their operations to others;

avoiding at the same time all attempts at subverting, by violence, established institutions, or outraging public sentiment by intemperate discussions. The doctrine now unfolded, if true, authorises us to predicate that the most successful method of ameliorating the condition of mankind, will be that which appeals most directly to their moral sentiments and intellect; and, I may add from experience and observation, that, in proportion as any individual becomes acquainted with the real constitution of the human mind, will his conviction of the efficacy of this method increase.

The next step ought to be to teach those laws to the young.* Their minds, not being pre-occupied by prejudices, will recognise them as congenial to their constitution; the first generation that has embraced them from infancy will proceed to modify the institutions of society into accordance with their dictates; and in the course of ages they may at length be acknowledged as practically useful. All *true* theories have ultimately been adopted and influenced practice; and I see no reason to fear that the present will prove an exception. The failure of all previous systems is the natural consequence of their being unfounded; if this one shall resemble them, it will deserve, and assuredly will meet with, a similar fate. A perception of the importance of the natural laws will lead to their observance, and this will be attended with an improved developement of brain, thereby increasing the desire and capacity for obedience.

Finally. If it be true that the Natural Laws must be obeyed as a preliminary condition to happiness in this world, and if virtue and happiness be inseparably allied, the religious instructers of mankind may probably discover

---

* Some observations on Education will be found in the Phrenological Journal, vol. iv. p. 407.

in the general and prevalent ignorance of these laws, one reason of the limited success which has hitherto attended their own efforts at improving the condition of mankind; and they may perhaps perceive it to be not inconsistent with their sacred office, to instruct men in the natural institutions of the Creator, in addition to his revealed will, and to recommend obedience to both. They exercise so vast an influence over the best members of society, that their countenance may hasten, or their opposition retard, by a century, the practical adoption of the natural laws, as guides of human conduct.

APPENDIX.

NOTE I.

NATURAL LAWS.—Text, p. 13.

In the text it is mentioned, that many philosophers have treated of the Laws of Nature. The following are examples :

Mr. Stewart says, ' To examine the economy of nature in the phenomena of the lower animals, and to compare their instincts with the physical circumstances of their external situation, forms one of the finest speculations of Natural History ; and yet it is a speculation to which the attention of the natural historian has seldom been directed. Not only Buffon, but Ray and Durham, have passed it over slightly ; nor, indeed, do I know of any one who has made it the object of a particular consideration but Lord Kames, in a short appendix to one of his sketches.'—*Elements of the Philosophy of the Human Mind*, vol. iii. p. 368.

Mr. Stewart also uses the following words :—' Numberless examples show that Nature has done no more for man than was necessary for his preservation, leaving him to make many acquisitions for himself, which she has imparted immediately to the brutes.

' My own idea is, as I have said on a different occasion, that both *instinct* and *experience* are here concerned, and that the share which belongs to each in producing the result, can be ascertained by an appeal to facts alone.'—Vol. iii. ch. 338.

Montesquieu introduces his Spirit of Laws by the following observations :—' Laws, in their most general signification, are the necessary relations derived from the nature of things. In this sense, all beings have their laws ; the Deity has his laws ; the material world its laws ; the intelligences superior to man have their laws ; the beasts their laws ; man his laws.

' Those who assert that *a blind fatality produced the various effects we behold in this world*, are guilty of a very great absurdity : for can any thing be more absurd than to pretend that a blind fatality could be productive of intelligent beings ?

'There is, then, a primitive reason; and laws are the relations which subsist between it and different beings, and the relations of these beings among themselves.

'God is related to the universe as creator and preserver; *the laws by which he has created all things are those by which he preserves them.* He acts according to these rules, because he knows them; he knows them because he made them; and he made them because they are relative to his wisdom and power, &c.

'Man, as a physical being, is, like other bodies, governed by invariable laws.'—Spirit of Laws, b. i. c. i.

Justice BLACKSTONE observes, that ' Law, in its most general and comprehensive sense, signifies a rule of action; and *is applied indiscriminately to all kinds of action, whether animate or inanimate, rational or irrational.* Thus we say, the laws of motion, of gravitation, of optics, or mechanics, as well as the laws of nature and of nations. Thus, when the Supreme Being formed the universe, and created matter out of nothing, he impressed certain *principles* upon that matter, from which it can never depart, and without which it would cease to be. When he put that matter into motion, he established *certain laws of motion,* to which all moveable bodies must conform.'—' If we farther advance from mere inactive matter to *vegetable and animal life,* WE SHALL FIND THEM STILL GOVERNED BY LAWS; more numerous, indeed, but *equally fixed and invariable.* The whole progress of plants, from the seed to the root, and from thence to the seed again;—the method of animal nutrition, digestion, secretion, and all other branches of vital economy;—are *not left to chance,* or the will of the creature itself, but are performed in a wondrous involuntary manner, and *guided by unerring rules laid down by the great Creator.* This, then, is the general signification of law, a rule of action dictated by some superior being; and in those creatures that have neither power to think, nor the will, such laws must be invariably obeyed, so long as the creature itself subsists; for its existence depends on that obedience.' *Blackstone's Commentaries on the Laws of England,* vol. i. sect. 2.

'The word *law,*' says Mr. Erskine, ' is frequently made use of, both by *divines and philosophers,* in a large acceptation, to express *the settled method of God's providence,* by which he preserves the order of the MATERIAL WORLD *in such a manner, that nothing in it may deviate from that uniform course which he has appointed for it.* And as brute matter is merely passive, without the least degree of choice upon its part, *these laws are* INVIOLABLY OBSERVED *in the material creation, every part of which continues to act, immutably, according to the rules that were from the beginning prescribed to it by infinite wisdom.* Thus philosophers have given the appellation of *law* to that motion which incessantly pervades and agitates the universe, and is ever changing the form and substance of things, dissolving some, and raising others, as from their ashes, to fill up the void : Yet so, that amidst all the fluctuations by which particular things are affected, the universe is still preserved without diminution. Thus also they speak of the *laws* of fluids, of gravitation, &c. and *the word is used, in this sense, in several passages of the sacred writings:* in the book of Job, and in Proverbs viii. 29, where God is said to have given *his law* to the seas that they should not pass his commandment.'—*Erskine's Institutes of the Laws of Scotland,* book i. tit. i. sect. 1.

Discussions about the Laws of Nature, rather than inquiries into them, were common in France, during the Revolution; and, having become associated, in imagination, with the crimes and horrors of that period, they continue to be regarded, by some individuals, as inconsistent with religion and morality. A coincidence between the views maintained in the preceding Essay, and a passage in VOLNEY, has been pointed out to me as an objection to the whole doctrine. VOLNEY's words are the following :—' It is a law of nature, that water flows from an upper to a lower situation ; that it seeks its level ; that it is heavier than air ; that all bodies tend towards the earth ; that flame rises towards the sky ; that it destroys the organization of vegetables and animals ; that air is essential to the life of certain animals ; that, in certain cases, water suffocates and kills them ; that certain juices of plants, and certain minerals, attack their organs, and destroy their life ;—and the same of a variety of facts.

' Now, since these facts, and many similar ones, are constant, regular, and immutable, they become so many real and positive commands, to which man is bound to conform, under the express penalty of punishment attached to their infraction, or well-being connected with their observance. So that if a man were to pretend to see clearly in the dark, or is regardless of the progress of the seasons, or the action of the elements ; if he pretends to exist under water, without drowning ; to handle fire without burning himself ; to deprive himself of air without suffocating ; or to drink poison without destroying himself ; he receives, for each infraction of the law of nature, a corporal punishment proportioned to his transgression. If, on the contrary, he observes these laws, and founds his practice on the precise and regular relation which they bear to him, he preserved his existence, and renders it as happy as it is capable of being rendered ; and since all these laws, considered in relation to the human species, have in view only one common end, that of their preservation and their happiness ; whence it has been agreed to assemble together the different ideas, and express them by a single word, and call them collectively by the name of the "*Law of Nature*."'—Volney's *Law of Nature*, 3d edit. pp. 21, 24.

I feel no embarrassment by this coincidence; but remark, first, That various authors, quoted in the text and in this note, advocated the importance of the laws of nature, long before the French Revolution was heard of; secondly, That the existence of the laws of nature is as obvious to the understanding, as the existence of the external world, and of the human mind and body themselves to the senses; thirdly, That these laws, being inherent in creation, must have proceeded from the Deity; fourthly, That if the Deity is powerful, just, and benevolent, they must harmonize with the constitution of man; and, lastly, That if the laws of nature have been instituted by the Deity, and been framed in wise, benevolent, and just relationship to the human constitution, they must at all times form the highest and most important subjects of human investigation, and remain altogether unaffected by the errors, follies, and crimes of those who endeavour to expound them; just as religion continues holy, venerable, and uncontaminated, notwithstanding the hypocrisy, wickedness, and inconsistency of individuals professing themselves her interpreters and friends.

That the views of the natural laws themselves, advocated in this Essay, are diametrically opposite to the practical conduct of the French revolutionary ruffians, requires no demonstration. My fundamental principle is, that man can enjoy happiness on earth only by placing his habitual conduct under the supremacy of the moral sentiments, and intellect, and that this is the *law of his nature*. No doctrine can be more opposed than this to fraud, robbery, blasphemy, and murder.

It may be urged, that all past speculations about the laws of nature have proved more imposing than useful; and that while the laws themselves afford materials for elevated declamation on the part of philosophers, they form no secure guides even to the learned, and much less to the illiterate, in practical conduct. In answer, I would respectfully repeat what has frequently been urged in the text, that, before we can discover the laws of nature, applicable to man, we must know, first, The constitution of man himself; secondly, The constitution of external nature; and, thirdly, We must compare the two. But, previous to the discovery of Phrenology, the mental constitution of man was a matter of vague conjecture, and endless debate; and the connexion between his mental powers and his organized system, was involved in the deepest obscurity. The brain, the most important organ of the body, had no ascertained functions. Before the introduction of this science, therefore, men were rather impressed with the unspeakable importance of a knowledge of the laws of nature, than acquainted with the laws themselves; and even the knowledge of the external world actually possessed, could not, in many instances, be rendered available, on account of its relationship to the qualities of man being unascertained, and unascertainable, so long as these qualities themselves were unknown.

Note II.

ORGANIC LAWS.—Text, p. 76.

It is a very common error, not only among philosophers, but among practical men, to imagine that the *feelings* of the mind are communicated to it through the medium of the *intellect ;* and, in particular, that if no indelicate objects reach the eyes, or expressions penetrate the ears, perfect purity will necessarily reign within the soul ; and, carrying this mistake into practice, they are prone to object to all discussion of the subjects treated of under the ' Organic Laws,' in works designed for general use. But their principle of reasoning is fallacious, and the practical result has been highly detrimental to society. The *feelings* have existence and activity distinct from the *intellect ;* they spur it on to obtain their own gratification ; and it may become either their slave or guide, according as it is enlightened concerning their constitution, and objects, and the laws of nature to which they are subjected. The most profound philosophers have inculcated this doctrine : and, by phrenological observation, it is demonstrably established. The organs of the feelings are distinct from those of the intellectual faculties; they are larger ; and, as each faculty, *cæteris paribus,* acts with a power proportionate to the size of its organ, the feelings are obviously the active or impelling powers. The cerebellum, or organ of Amativeness, is the largest of the whole mental organs ; and, being endowed with natural activity, it fills the mind spontaneously with emotions and suggestions which may be directed, controlled, and resisted, in outward manifestation, by intellect and moral sentiment, but which cannot be prevented from arising, nor eradicated after they exist. The whole question, therefore, resolves itself into this, Whether it is most beneficial to enlighten and direct that feeling, or (under the influence of an error in philosophy, and false delicacy founded on it,) to permit it to riot in all the fierceness of a blind animal instinct, withdrawn from the eye of reason, but not thereby deprived of its vehemence and importunity. The former course appears to me to be the only one consistent with reason and morality; and I have adopted it in reliance on the good sense of my readers, that they will at once discriminate between practical instruction concerning this feeling, addressed to the intellect, and lascivious representations addressed to the mere propensity itself; with the latter of which the enemies of all improvement may attempt to confound my observations. Every function of the mind and body is instituted by the Creator; all may be abused; and it is impossible regularly to avoid abuse of them, except by being instructed in their nature, objects, and relations. This instruction ought to be addressed exclusively to the intellect; and, when it is so, it is science of the most beneficial description. The propriety, nay necessity, of acting on this principle, becomes more and more apparent, when it is considered that the discussions of the text suggest only intellectual ideas to individuals in whom the feeling in question is naturally weak, and that such minds perceive no indelicacy in knowledge which is calculated to be useful; while, on the other hand, persons in whom the feeling is naturally strong, are precisely those who stand in need of direction, and to whom, of all others, instruction is the most necessary.

Fortified by these observations, I venture to record some additional facts communicated by persons on whose accuracy reliance may be placed.

A gentleman, who has paid much attention to the rearing of horses, informed me, that the male racehorse, when excited, but not exhausted, by running, has been found by experience, to be in a most favourable condition for transmitting swiftness and vivacity to his offspring. Another gentleman stated, that he was himself present when the pale gray color of a male horse was objected to; that the groom thereupon presented before the eyes of the male another female from the stable, of a very particular, but pleasing, variety of colours, asserting that the latter would determine the complexion of the offspring; and that in point of fact it did so. The experiment was tried in the case of a second female, and the result was so completely the same, that the two young horses, in point of colour, could scarcely be distinguished, although their spots were extremely uncommon. The account of Laban and the peeled rods laid before the cattle to produce spotted calves, is an example of the same kind.

PORTAL mentions the hereditary descent of blindness and deafness. His words are: 'MORGAGNI has seen three sisters dumb *" d'origine."* Other authors also cite examples, and I have seen like cases myself.' In a note, he adds, ' I have seen three children out of four of the same family blind from birth by amaurosis, or gutta serena.—*Portal, Memoires sur Plusieurs Maladies*, tome iii. p. 193. Paris, 1808.

In the Quarterly Journal of Agriculture, No. I., there are several valuable articles illustrative of the Organic Laws in the inferior animals. I select the following examples:

' Every one knows that the hen of any bird will lay eggs although no male be permitted to come near her; and that those eggs are only wanting in the vital principle which the impregnation of the male conveys to them. Here, then, we see the female able to make an egg, with yolk and white, shell and every part, just as it ought to be, so that we might at the first glance, suppose that here, at all events, the female has the greatest influence. But see the change which the male produces. Put a Bantam cock to a large sized hen and she will instantly lay a small egg; the chick will be short, in the leg, have feathers to the foot, and put on the appearance of the cock; so that it is a frequent complaint where Bantams are kept, that they make the hens lay small eggs, and spoil the breed. Reverse the case; put a large dunghill cock to Bantam hens, and instantly they will lay larger eggs, and the chicks will be good-sized birds, and the Bantam will have nearly disappeared. Here, then, are a number of facts known to every one, or at least open to be known by every one, clearly proving the influence of the male in some animals; and as I hold it to be an axiom that nature never acts by contraries, never outrages the law clearly fixed in one species, by adopting the opposite course in another,—therefore as in the case of an equilateral triangle on the length of one side being given we can with certainty demonstrate that of the remaining; so, having found these laws to exist in one race of animals, we are entitled to assume that every species is subjected to the self same rules,—the whole bearing, in fact, the same relation to each other as the radii of a circle.'

' *A method of obtaining a greater number of One Sex, at the option of the Proprietor, in the Breeding of Live Stock.*—Extracted from the Quarterly Journal of Agriculture, No. I. p. 63.

In the Annales de l'Agriculture Français, vols. 37 and 38, some very interesting experiments are recorded, which have lately been made in France, on the Breeding of Live Stock. M. Charles Girou de Buzareingues proposed, at a meeting of the Agricultural Society of Severac, on the 3d of July, 1826, to divide a flock of sheep into two equal parts, so that a greater number of males or females, at the choice of the proprietor, should be produced from each of them. Two of the members of the Society offered their flocks to become the subjects of his experiments, and the results have now been communicated, which are in accordance with the author's expectations.

'The first experiment was conducted in the following manner: He recommended very young rams to be put to the flock of ewes, from which the proprietor wished the greater number of females in their offspring; and also, that, during the season when the rams were with the ewes, they should have more abundant pasture than the other; while, to the flock from which the proprietor wished to obtain male lambs chiefly, he recommended him to put strong and vigorous rams four or five years old. The following tabular view contains the result of this experiment.

FLOCK FOR FEMALE LAMBS.

Age of the Mothers.	Sex of the Lambs.	
	Males.	Females.
Two years,	14	26
Three years,	16	29
Four years,	5	21
Total,	35	76
Five years and older,	18	8
Total,	53	84

N. B.—There were three twin births in this flock. Two rams served it, one fifteen months, the other nearly two years old.

FLOCK FOR MALE LAMBS.

Age of the Mothers.	Sex of the Lambs.	
	Males.	Females.
Two years,	7	3
Three years,	15	14
Four years,	33	14
Total,	55	31
Five years and older,	25	24
Total,	80	55

N. B.—There were no twin births in this flock. Two strong rams, one four, the other five years old, served it.

'The second experiment is thus related by the author:

'During the summer of 1826, M. Cournuejouls, kept upon a very dry pasture, belonging to the village of Bez, a flock of 106 ewes, of which 84 belonged to himself, and 22 to his shepherds. Towards the end of October, he divided his flock into two sections, of 42 heads each, the one composed of the strongest ewes, from four to five years old; the other of the weakest beasts under four or above five years old. The first was destined to produce a greater number of females than the second. After it was marked with pitch in my presence, it was taken to much better pasture behind Panouse, where it was delivered to four male lambs, about six months old, and of good promise. The second remained upon the pasture of Bez, and was served by two strong rams, more than three years old.

'The ewes belonging to the shepherds, which I shall consider as forming a third section, and which are in general stronger and better fed than those of the master, because their owners are not always particular in preventing them from trespassing on the cultivated lands, which are not enclosed, were mixed with those of the second flock, the result was, that the

	Males.	Females
First Section gave,	15	25
The Second,	26	14
The Third,	10	12
In the First Section there were Two Twin Births,	0	4
In the Second and Third there were also Two,	3	1

" Besides these very decisive experiments, M. Girou relates some others, made with horses and cattle, in which his success in producing a greater number of one sex rather than another also appears. The general law, as far as we are able to detect it, seems to be, that, when animals are in good condition, plentifully supplied with food, and kept from breeding as fast as they might do, they are most likely to produce females. Or, in other words, when a race of animals is in circumstances favourable for its increase, nature produces the greatest number of that sex which, in animals that do not pair, is most efficient for increasing the numbers of the race: But, if they are in a bad climate, or on stinted pasture, or, if they have already given birth to a numerous offspring, then nature, setting limits to the increase of the race, produces more males than females. Yet, perhaps it may be premature to attempt to deduce any law from experiments which have not yet been sufficiently extended. M. Girou is dispsoed to ascribe much of the effect to the age of the ram, independent of the condition of the ewe."

Note III.

DEATH.—Text, p. 128.

The decreasing Mortality of England is strikingly supported by the following extract from the Scotsman of 16th April, 1828. It is well known that this paper is edited by Mr. Charles Maclaren, a gentleman whose extensive information, and scrupulous regard to accuracy and truth, stamp the highest value on his statements of fact: and whose profound and comprehensive intellect warrants a well-grounded reliance on his philosophical conclusions.

"DIMINISHED MORTALITY IN ENGLAND. The diminution of the annual mortality in England amidst an alleged increase of crime, misery, and pauperism, is an extraordinary and startling fact, which merits a more careful investigation than it has received. We have not time to go deeply into the subject: but we shall offer a remark or two on the question, how the apparent annual mortality is effected by the introduction of the cow-pox, and the stationary or progressive state of the population. In 1780, according to Mr. RICK-MAN, the annual deaths were 1 in 40, or *one-fortieth* part of the population died every year; in 1821, the proportion was 1 in 58. It follows, that, out of any given number of persons, 1000 or 10,000, scarcely more than two deaths take place now for three that took place in 1780, or the mortality has diminished 45 per cent. The parochial registers of burials in England, from which this statement is derived, are known to be incorrect, but as they continue to be kept without alteration in the same way, the errors of one year, are justly conceived to balance those of another, and they thus afford *comparative* results upon which considerable reliance may be placed.

"A community is made up of persons of many various ages, among whom the law of mortality is very different. Thus, according to the Swedish tables, the deaths among children from the moment of birth up to 10 years of age, are 1 in 22 per annum; from 10 to 20, the deaths are only 1 in 185. Among the old again, mortality is of course great. From 70 to 80, the deaths are 1 in 9; from 80 to 90, they are 1 in 4. Now, a community like that of New York or Ohio, where marriages are made early, and the births are numerous, necessarily contains a large proportion of young persons, among whom the proportional mortality is low, and a small proportion of the old who die off rapidly. A community in which the births are numerous, is like a regiment receiving a vast number of young and healthy recruits, and in which, of course, as a whole, the annual deaths will be few compared with those in another regiment chiefly filled with veterans, though among the persons at any particular age, such as 20, 40, or 50, the mortality will be as great in the one regiment as the other. It may thus happen, that the annual mortality among 1000 persons in Ohio, may be considerably less than in France, while the *Expectation of Life*, or the chance which an individual has to reach to a certain age, may be no greater in the former country than in the latter; and hence we see that a diminution in the rate of mortality is not a certain proof of an increase in the value of life, or an improvement in the condition of the people.

'But the effect produced by an increased number of births is less than might be imagined, owing to the very great mortality among infants in the first year of their age. Not having time for the calculations necessary to get at the precise result, which are pretty complex, we avail ourselves of some statements given by Mr. MILNE in his work on Annuities. Taking the Swedish tables as a basis, and supposing the law of mortality to remain the same for each period of life, he has compared the proportional number of deaths in a population which is stationary, and in one which increases 15 per cent. in 20 years. The result is, that when the mortality in the stationary society is *one* in 36.13, that in the progressive society is one in 37.33, a difference equal to 3¼ per cent. Now, the population of England and Wales inrceased 34.3 per cent. in the 20 years ending in 1821, but in the interval from 1811 to 1821, the rate was equivalent to 39¼ per cent. upon 20 years; and the apparent diminution of mortality arising from this circumstance must of course have been about 8¼ per cent. We are assuming, however, that the population was absolutely stationary at 180, which was not the case. According to Mr. MILNE (p. 437,) the average annual increase in the five years ending 1784, was 1 in 155; in the ten years ending 1821, according to the census, it was 1 in 60. Deducting, then, the proportional part corresponding to the former, which is 3¼, there remains 5¼. If Mr. MILNE's tables, therefore, are correct, *we may infer that the progressive state of the population causes a diminution of* 5¼ *per cent. in the annual mortality*—a diminution which is only *apparent*, because it arises entirely from the great proportion of births, and is not accompanied with any real increase in the value of human life.

' A much greater change—not apparent but real—was produced by the introduction of the vaccination in 1798. It was computed, that, in 1795, when the population of the British Isles was 15,000,-000, the deaths produced by the small-pox amounted to 36,000, or nearly 11 per cent. of the whole annual mortality. (See article *Vaccination* in the Supplement to Encyclopedia Britannica, p. 713.) Now, since not more than one case in 330 terminates fatally under the cow-pox system, either directly by the primary infection, or from the other disease supervening : the whole of the young persons destroyed by the small pox might be considered as saved, were vaccination universal, and always properly performed. This is not precisely the case, but one or one and a-half per cent. will cover the deficiencies; and we may therefore conclude, that *vaccination has diminished the annual mortality fully nine per cent.* After we had arrived at this conclusion by the process described, we found it confirmed by the authority of Mr. MILNE, who estimates in a note to one of his tables, that the mortality of 1 in 40 would be diminished to 1 in 43—5, by exterminating small-pox. Now, this is almost precisely 9 per cent.

'We stated, that the diminution of the annual mortality between 1780 and 1821 was 45 per cent., according to Mr. RICKMAN. If we deduct from this 9 per cent. for the effect of vaccination, and 5 per cent. as only apparent, resulting from the increasing proportion of births—31 per cent. remains, *which we apprehend, can only be accounted for by an improvement in the habits, morals, and physical condition of the people.* Independently, then, of the two causes alluded to, the value of human life since 1780, has increased in a ratio which would diminish the annual mortality from 1 in 40 to 1 in 52½, a fact which is indisputably of great importance, and worth volumes of declamation in illustrating the true situation of the labouring classes. We have founded our conclusion on data derived entirely from English returns; but there is no doubt that it applies equally to Scotland. It is consoling to find, from this very unexceptionable species of evidence, that though there is much privation and suffering in the country, the situation of the people has been, on the whole, progressively improving during the last forty years. But how much greater would the advance have been, had they been less taxed, and better treated? and how much room is there still for future melioration, by spreading instruction, amending our laws, lessening the temptations to crime, and improving the means of correction and reform? In the mean time, it ought to be some encouragement to philanthropy to learn, that it has not to struggle against invincible obstacles, and that even when the prospect was least cheering to the eye, its efforts were silently benefiting society.'

It has been mentioned to me, that the late Dr. MONRO, in his anatomical lectures, stated, that, as far as he could observe, the human body, as a machine, was perfect,—that it bore within itself no marks by which we could possibly predicate its decay,—that it was apparently calculated to go on forever,—and that we learned only by experience that it would not do so; and some persons have conceived this to be an authority against the doctrine maintained in Chap. III. Sect. 2. that death is apparently inherent in organization. In answer, I beg to observe, that if we were to look at the sun only for one moment of time, say at noon, no circumstance, in its appearance, would indicate that it had ever risen, or that it would ever set; but, if we had traced its progress from the horizon to the meridian, and down again till the long shadows of evening prevailed, we should have ample grounds for inferring, that, if the same causes that had produced these changes continued to operate, it would undoubtedly at length disappear. In the same way, if we were to confine our observations on the human body to a mere point of time, it is certain that, from the appearances of that moment, we could not infer that it had grown up, by gradual increase, or that it would decay; but this is the case only, because our faculties are not fitted to penetrate into the essential nature and dependencies of things. Any man, who had seen the body decrease in old age, could, without hesitation, predicate, that, if the same causes which had produced that effect went on operating, dissolution would at last inevitably occur; and if his Causality were well developed, he would not hesitate to say that a *cause* of the decrease and dissolution must exist, although he could not tell by examining the body what it was. By analysing alcohol, no person could predicate, independently of experience, that it would produce intoxication; and, nevertheless, there must be a cause in the constitution of the alcohol, in that of the body, and in the relationship between them, why it produces this effect. The notion, therefore, of Dr. Monro, does not prove that death is not an essential law of organization, but only that the human faculties are not able, by dissection, to discover that the cause of it is inherent in the bodily constitution itself. It does not follow, however, that this inference may not be legitimately drawn from phenomena collected from the whole period of corporeal existence.

Note IV.

INFRINGEMENT OF THE MORAL LAWS.—Text, p. 159.

The deterioration of the operative classes of Britain which I attribute to excessive labour, joined with great alterations of high and low wages, and occasionally with absolute idleness and want, is illustrated by the following extracts:—

'Unemployed Weavers in Lanarkshire. On Saturday last, a meeting of weavers' delegates from the various districts in this neighbourhood, was held in the usual place. The object of the meeting was to receive from the several districts an account of the number of weavers out of employment, which statement it was intended to lay before the Lord Provost and Magistrates. The following are the returns given in:—Anderston contains 708 looms, of which 386 are idle. Baillieston-toll contains 150 looms, of these 98 are empty. The district of north Bridgeton contains, in whole, between 400 and 500 looms. The returns are only from about one half of this district, which contains 150 empty looms. For the centre and south districts of Bridgeton, the accounts are incomplete.

In the former 180, and in the latter 60, empty looms were taken up. In Charleston there are 132 idle. In Cowcaddens, of 300 looms, 120 are idle. In Clyde, Bell, and Tobago Streets, of about 500 looms, there are 74 idle; and 100 working webs which cannot average 8d. a-day. In drygate, there are 105 idle; in Drygate-toll 73; in Duke Street 18. In Gorbals, containing 365 looms, there are 223 idle. In Havannah, out of 130 looms, there are 48 idle. In the district of Keppoch-hill, of 70 weavers, there are 20 idle. The district of King Street is divided into ten wards; returns are only given in from four, which contain 70 empty looms. In Pollockshaws, containing about 800 looms, there are 216 idle. In Rutherglen there are 167 idle. In Springbank, of 141 weavers, there are 58 unemployed; and in Strathbungo, containing 104 looms, there are 28 idle, 25 of whom are married men. Parkhead, Camlachie and some other extensive districts, have not yet given in their returns. The delegates, before separating, appointed a general meeting to be held in the Green this day, to decide upon an address to the Magistrates, requesting them to endeavour to procure employment for the idle hands.'—*Glasgow Chronicle, Tuesday, March,* 1826.

'SHEEP TRADE. The late commercial crisis, like a death blow, has paralyzed the whole activity of the country, and left scarcely a single branch of its trade and industry unscathed. It was at first fondly hoped that the storm would pass without such remote districts as our own having much reason to complain of its visitation; but nothing, as the present instance proves, is more certain than that the distresses of the commercial, must also in all cases be more or less felt by the agricultural classes of the community. The demand for wool has now so far ceased as to operate most injuriously upon the price of sheep, which cannot presently be sold but at a very considerable loss to the farmer. In the latter part, or "back season," as it is called, of 1824, black-faced ewes—their example applies equally to the other kinds—were bought in for wintering at from 8s. to 12s. a-head; and, in the spring of 1825, immediately before lambing-time, these were disposed of in the English markets at so great a profit, that every farmer who could at all enter into the speculation, bought up at the end of the ensuing harvest, as much of that description of stock as his quantity of keep would seasonably permit. The number of sheep over those of the preceding year which were bought up for this purpose, may be judged of from the fact, that the highest inlay price of 1824 was the lowest of 1825— the rate for the latter year being, for black-faced ewes, from 12s. to 18s. But the present crisis came,—the manufacturers of England were obliged to retrench at meals in the article of mutton,—the de-

mand on the part of the butchers consequently ceased; and now those sheep which were purchased at so extravagant a rate, are necessarily sold, upon an average, at a loss of 2s. a-head upon the inlay price, without at all estimating the expense of keep. We know one extensive moorland farmer, who calculates upon loosing two hundred pounds in the present year from this cause alone, besides a vast loss which he must also sustain in consequence of the reduced price of wool. This cessation of demand in England was unfortunately not fully ascertained until several droves of lambing ewes had been despatched to that quarter; and the embarrassment of those who are placed in this predicament is the more afflicting, as their knowledge has been acquired too late to allow their availing themselves of the house of Muir, and other northern markets.'
— *Dumfries Courier, March*, 1826.

' *Details upon the Subject of Weavers' Wages, from the last Report of Emigration extracted from the Scotsman Newspaper, of* 10*th November*, 1827.

' Joseph Foster, a weaver, and one of the deputies of an emigration society in Glasgow, states that the labour is all paid by the piece; the hours of working are various, sometimes eighteen or nineteen out of twenty-four, and even all night once or twice a-week; and that the wages made by such labour, after deducting the necessary expenses, will not amount to more than from 4s. 6d. to 7s. per. week, some kinds of work paying better than others. When he commenced working as a weaver, from 1800 to 1805, the same amount of labour that now yields 4s. 6d. or 5s. would have yielded 20s. There are about 11,000 hand-looms going in Glasgow and its suburbs, some of which are worked by boys and girls, and he estimates the average net earnings of each hand-weaver at 5s. 6d. The principal subsistence of the weavers is oatmeal and potatoes, with occasionally some salt herring.

' Major Thomas Moodie, who had made careful inquiries into the state of the poor at Manchester, states, that the calico and other light plain work at Bolton and Blackburn, yields the weaver from 4s. to 5s. per week, by fourteen hours of daily labour. In the power-loom work, one man attends two looms, and earns from 7s. 6d. to 14s. per. week, according to the fineness of the Work. He understood that during the last ten years, weavers' wages had fallen on an average about 15s. per week.

' Mr. Thomas Hunton, manufacturer, Carlisle, states, that there are in Carlisle and its neighbourhood about 5500 families, or from 18,000 to 20,000 persons dependent on weaving. They are all hand-weavers, and are now in a very depressed state, in consequence of the increase of power-loom and factory weaving* in Manchester and elsewhere. Taking fifteen of his men, he finds that five of them, who are employed on the best work, had earned 5s. 6d. per week for the preceding month, deducting the necessary expenses of loom-rent, candles, tackling, &c.; the next five, who are upon work of the second quality, earned 3s. 11d.; and the third five earned 3s. 7½d. per week. They work from fourteen to sixteen hours a-day, and live chiefly on patatoes, butter-milk, and herrings.

'Mr. W. H. Hyett, Secretary to the Charity Committee in London, gives a detailed statement, to show, that, in the Hundred of Blackburn, comprising a population of 150,000 persons, 90,000 were out of employment in 1826! In April last, when he gave his evidence before the Committee, these persons had generally found work again, but at very low wages. They were labouring from twelve to fourteen hours a-day, and gaining from 4s. to 5s. 6d. per week.'

"Poor Rates, 28th March, 1828.—A document of great importance, though of a description by no means cheering, has been presented to the House of Commons,—the annual Abstract of the Returns of the Poor Rates levied and expended, with comparisons, showing the increase or diminution. The accounts show the expenditure of the year ending 25th March, 1827, compared with the previous year. The total sum levied in all the counties of England and Wales, in the last year, was £7,489,694; the sum expended for the relief of the poor, £6,179,877. The increase in that year throughout the whole of England and Wales, is nine per cent.; nine per cent. in one year on the whole sum expended. It is true that this is in part to be accounted for by the temporary distress of the manufacturing districts. (In Lancaster, the increase was forty-seven, the West Riding of York, thirty-one per cent.); but we are sorry to find, that in only three counties of England was there any the most trifling diminution. In Berks two, Hampshire five, Suffolk four per cent. The poor rates in England, therefore, amount to nearly double the whole landed rental of Scotland."

"*Extract from the Lord-Advocate's Speech in the House of Commons, 11th March, 1828, on the additional Circuit Court of Glasgow.*

"The Lord-Advocate, in rising to move for leave to bring in a bill to 'authorize an additional Court of Justiciary to be held at

---

* In what is called factory-weaving, an improved species of hand-loom is employed, in which the dressing and preparation of the web is effected by machinery, and the weaver merely sits and drives the shuttle.

Glasgow, and to facilitate criminal trial in Scotland,' said he did not anticipate any opposition to the motion. A great deal had been said of the progress of crime in this country, but he was sorry to say crime in Scotland had kept pace with that increase. A return had been made of the number of criminal commitments in each year, so far back as the year 1805. In that year the number of criminal commitments for all Scotland amounted only to 85. In 1809 it had risen to between 200 and 300; in 1819–20, it had increased to 400; and by the last return, it appeared, that, in 1827, 661 persons had been committed for trial. He was inclined to think, that the great increase of crime, particularly in the west of Scotland, was attributable, in no small degree, to the number of Irish who daily and weekly arrived there. He did not mean to say that the Irish themselves were in the habit of committing more crime than their neighbours; but he was of opinion, that their numbers tended to reduce the price of labour, and that an increase of crime was the consequence. Another cause was the great disregard manifested by parents for the moral education of their children. Formerly, the people of Scotland were remarkable for the paternal care which they took of their offspring. That had ceased in many instances to be the case. Not only were parents found who did not pay attention to the welfare of their children, but who were actually parties to their criminal pursuits, and participated in the fruits of their unlawful proceedings. When crime was thus on the increase, it was necessary to take measures for its speedy punishment. The great city of Glasgow, which contained 150,000 inhabitants, and to which his proposed measure was meant chiefly to apply, stood greatly in need of some additional jurisdiction. This would appear evident, when it was considered that the court which met there for the trial of capital offences, had also to act in the districts of Renfrew, Lanark, and Dunbarton. In 1812, the whole number of criminals tried in Glasgow was only 31; in 1820, it was 83; in 1823, it was 85; and in 1827, 211.—The learned lord concluded by moving for leave to bring in a bill to authorize an additional circuit court of justiciary to be held at Glasgow, and to facilitate trial in Scotland."

THE END.